EDDIE J. POWELL

MEDICAL MAFIA

TO

MODERN MARX

based on a true story

i

A childhood of many separate challenges from many state failures by the Irish establishment has led me to a life of taking my power back and not fitting into the current models within the establishment and instead find alternatives that remodel a far better establishment for all Longterm which is what living is all about standing out and overcoming rather than fitting in and staying in line.

DEDICATION

Caution to do with pushing far too many prescriptions that cause harm and death to many and will only continue until it is corrected. Pharma is now the very same model as big tobacco was before it was caught and sued for 240 plus billion for causing addictions and marketing to all ages making them customers for life. Pharma is worse than big tobacco because it boasts itself as a healthcare model and it would be out of business if everyone was healthy and the ones taking all the risks and responsibility here are the patients but they are made think they have to take all these drugs yet these drugs are exactly what could be making them far more ill than they were before their first prescription.

Brief Introduction

My name is Eddie Powell, and I would like to tell my personal story. It is a terrifying and powerful journey involving many frustrating conditions I was in due to my country being run by immoral systems. They were a little isolated with the condition I was given to live with throughout my childhood. I would like to add that all the names of doctors, hospitals, public houses, and the people I met throughout this journey have been made anonymous, but the cities and towns have been mentioned because they made the journey more meaningful with all their separate characteristics and are all large enough places to be freely spoken about.

I fought a common neurological condition, which has finally been labeled as left temporal lobe epilepsy, starting in 1981, for over twenty years. I didn't care I had it until I realized the fact that it was not acceptable in society and that we were a very much fully catholic country at the time. The catholic church said a lot of negative things about people with neurological conditions, which made life more difficult to live than actually having the condition in the first place.

I did, to a point, pity myself at first, since I was treated as if I were a second or third-class citizen. I related to people who migrate to other developed countries because they have to and feel hard done by due to leaving their home country or fleeing from war or Third World countries for a better life. I was in the same situation at home with the society in my own country.

This led to incredible anger and disappointment because of what I had. I think it was only because the country itself was going through a hard time too, being in a very deep recession that began in 1986, with a debt worse than Ethiopia at the time. But it was not I that caused that recession to happen, so the problem was not only that what I had was not fully accepted in the culture but the generation which was grown up had wrecked the country financially. People like me, who were seen as nobodies or burdens because of what we had, were their way of focusing on something else rather than their problems. Even though, without people like me who had a condition, so many doctors, scientists, pharmacists, and so on would be out of a job as sickness is why they have a job to survive in this world. My part was to, hopefully, get cured one day of what I had.

I felt I was a target due to what I had for people who were not happy with their positions in society, so they were attracted to seeing more faults in others and stayed ignorant and arrogant about their problems. This is the same as people targeting people who have good times. And the cycle goes on and on, consisting of people covering up their big personal issues, the gap between the rich and poor, the differences between men and women, the separate beliefs in religion, etc.

But in the end, I realized looking for a position in a backward society that wrecked the country financially was the wrong road to take because it would mean that I would be one of those who think they are free but are complete slaves in an engineered system.

My attitude grew with how I was treated. I became less fearful of anyone who came near me, became more daring because I had something I was not able to control, less lonesome as I saw just as many faults in society as they saw in me. I was more ambitious to go on full-force with my destiny because I was not, and did not want to be, the same as everybody else in a massive system that was just a bubble.

Because, as your ego can only bring you so far, I thought it's the same with being in a system. I also saw that they make you think you have to go this way or else, which is how people let their whole lives be controlled by fear and not by love, hope, faith, self-belief, or self-control. For someone in my condition, who already felt controlled to a certain extent, having to take medications every day or else get a seizure, really set me free from being conditioned to other bigger systems.

So, considering the fact I was already in a have-to condition with some things or others, I questioned other things that people thought they have to do or be but don't have to at all! I was able to understand people and what kind of self-destruction their ignorance was creating, which — in my mind — would surpass any illness or hardship because look at the word (ignorance), they're ignoring other possibilities that could be better or worse.

I will explain how I learned about life, emotionally and financially, without the full support of the systems, and the mistakes I saw in them since I felt that I was not fully accepted in them anyway, which is what set me free to create my des-tiny. But because I was living in the real world where an illness makes you learn from the heart rather than the conscious mind, and in some ways, it can make you learn much faster emotionally, I found my paths to work on and respected myself. But I also became self-destructive in many bad times, when I felt like giving up or isolating myself from other people and destructive medical and educational systems.

So, at the age of four, in 1985, when Ireland was in a very deep recession — hitting a worse debt rate than Ethiopia — I was in my room playing just like any normal kid. I probably felt the vibe of the pressure people were under since a child's intuition is higher, but with no understanding of it, I was sitting on the floor, playing with cars as a normal boy would do. Then, all of a sudden, my temperature went from normal to high, and my eyes began to roll up my forehead as I became unconscious. I started to go purple, as my temperature became cold. The next thing I knew, I had a bad tantrum and started jerking and had a grand mal seizure. So, my parents wrapped me up in a blanket and brought me to Cork Medical Hospital. The doctors did some tests on me. My mother instantly knew, due to her instincts, that it was, more than likely, a type of epilepsy. Her brother also grew up with the same illness but a different and less severe type of it and later grew out of it when he became an adult.

However, they didn't diagnose me with it right away and said it might have just been a once-off seizure, sending me home again a few days later. So, I was brought home, but later I, unfortunately, started getting several more grand mal seizures that lasted nearly five minutes or more. The doctors were doing more and more tests, such as CAT scans, and could not find the cause. They ruled out epilepsy, again.

My parents stood by, all day and night, frightened of what was going on. My mother was so frightened that she would not leave the room and my father was being strong by telling her, "Everything will be okay and we will get through whatever happens. There's a way around everything."

The doctors warned my parents that if I didn't come around soon, I could end up being brain-damaged, so they should be prepared for the worst scenario.

Shortly after coming around and waking up, I was diagnosed with epilepsy, but there was no name for what type of it I had as there are numerous types of epilepsy today. So, like my mum presumed at first and was right, it was temporal lobe epilepsy, which was not known until I was around twenty.

When I was young, I found it easy enough to live with, being young, daring, and stupid. I didn't give a damn about having it because I had it from the start. I just gave a damn that it was treated with incredible negativity. Since this was happening, I did even more daring things than an adult did, just to show people that I was not a disabled child because I got seizures. It is no different to people who get drunk each weekend and don't know where they were when they were drunk and turn around and say they had a great night yet can't remember much of it, and the hangover is self-inflicted.

However, trying to keep this attitude up constantly, when the economy is on a downturn, is like trying to change the country all at once or going against the tide and getting caught in the current of it, going around in circles. And it can bring a fit of anger or an episode of depression to those who put such pressure on themselves. I was as wild as any other child and didn't spend my time worrying if I'd have a seizure at all. I just accepted I had it but didn't accept it was going to dictate me and certainly not condition me. No way was I going there even though I had an incredible fear that later in life, I could be locked up if it still wasn't acceptable in socie-ties and that I might not get a job with it, etc.

The anxiety had made me think for myself since a very young age and do a lot of things opposite to what most people do as they grow up. This made me even more skeptical, being aware and questioning everything twice rather than just going with a system. To a degree, I gained self-independence with this attitude, same as countries have, in history, gained independence from empires by creating their systems. I was doing all the things like any normal kid would, such as climbing, running, and getting up to no good. But all kids do not obey everything, especially if they have a point to prove. I was not going to hang around self-pitying until someday I might be cured or whatever. That was an attitude I knew would not last, so I grew out of it pretty quickly.

It was more difficult for my parents at that stage as they did all the worrying and didn't know how to treat me. They had four other children to care for and keep a roof over their heads. But, as I said earlier, I was not being dictated by anyone. I promised myself that the more someone tried to dictate me because I got seizures, the more independence I would gain for myself, no matter how hard it became.

It wasn't that I was a bad child. It was to show that people with so-called disabilities, or whatever people want to label them with, can do the same things as people who don't have them. I wanted to simply go to any level to make that point, hoping that others with any type of disability will also fight against the ignorance and arrogance of systems and society.

It's just that they have more of a challenge ahead of them. They should be allowed to deal with it since whatever they do does not harm others. Society has way more illnesses and diseases of its own, especially bipolar disease, with all the ups and downs it creates.

Epilepsy is just a condition that was treated with such an over-the-top negative response, with more drama than acceptance, and if drunkenness was treated just as bad as it was, then we would probably have a sober society in no time. Many people cope with it perfectly well and some people who made history had it, such as Julius Caesar and Neil Young. It's not as if it is anything new to fear as it is very much known as the sacred disease. Certain medications for some people can threaten them with very few side effects and many can stay seizure-free.

I believe from experience that a lot about being cured is also up to the individual, and many of us can do impossible things with our life if we put ourselves to the challenge. It's not something that requires you to live a different life with if you're daring enough to prove yourself to others that you're no different than any other person.

In Ireland, one in every 110 people has epilepsy. All the things you're not allowed because of having it can be quite a burden to live with. You may as well lie down if you're expected to obey everything because freedom is an expression and people with any condition are still human and labeling them as second or third class will provoke war within the people themselves to prove everyone wrong.

You're not meant to do certain things while living with it, which I found to be humiliating because we're all humans and nobody, whatever color, country, or belief they have, should ever be treated as second-class. Only the people who control those systems and make a profit from others suffering should be labeled as second-class and psychotic.

No one in the world can expect everyone to be on the same level when the big question is why are we here? And how did we get here? People with epilepsy can work hard too. Very hard. The last thing they want to hear is people gossiping about their problem, feeling sorry for them, wishing they could get better.

To some people, that may sound as if they're only trying to help, but gossiping is the last thing that helps. Gossiping makes people lose control of their destiny and lose their dignity, depending on what it's about. It certainly doesn't do anyone a favor. Where is it going to get the person with the problem, hearing other people going on about their problem, talking to people whom the person with the problem doesn't even know? Nowhere! It is just going to make them feel worse and try and run a mile from those types of people, hoping there might be a cure for gossiping too and feeling isolated from the rest.

Pitying someone is useless, no matter what's wrong with them. We all need to be given dignity before any sympathy. Being there for them and telling them something you have been through will be the start of a conversation that you would never think you could experience. Nothing is more helpful than two people having a heart-to-heart conversation, bringing both minds back to neutral, which is the natural system that we can all maintain.

Warnings, also known as auras, came before every seizure. I had many different types of them from the age of five to eleven□the aura I'd get before a seizure was like the start of a panic attack or anxiety attack. At first, you'd feel your body beginning to strain from the bottom up and, suddenly, an im-age appears that the ground is starting to break up and there's a fire underneath. This, had a lot to do with an overactive imagination, thinking I was condemned to hell since I had this illness and knowing that, in history, people thought it was from the devil.

It was feeling as if I was about to fall into hell, and by the time I fell unconscious, the seizure began. Some of these were also the side-effects of some drugs and the rest had to do with the over-active imagination or feeling of anxiety.

From the age of eleven to eighteen, I would start moving my tongue as if I was tasting something off and get this weird pulse coming up my stomach that started from the heart and moved up towards the eyes. That's when I would start moving my tongue more as if I was going to get sick or the taste was just becoming unbearable and then, as the feeling moved up, I would start moving my left hand, roll my eyes up into my head, have the seizure and come around after it, sometimes on the ground. Other times, I could be in the ditch, etc., but whatever the case, I was not hiding behind closed doors because I fell often and got seizures, since I got right back up again and carried on.

I refused to ever lower myself to that standard of living. No other person with any other form of challenge to live through should ever allow it to dictate their life either. They should fight it like an enemy rather than getting to know it more. They should never allow it to overtake their life if it's stopping them from doing what they want to do.

From the age of nineteen to twenty-three, the final aura I was getting was sort of similar to the last. In this case, however, when the strange feeling was coming up from the base of my stomach, I would try to keep talking to myself to fight it off. This is the reason people can't tell others that they are about to have a seizure. This is all in the span of five to ten seconds. All of a sudden, the more you talk, the faster it comes as your pronunciation then goes. Then, all of a sudden, you have the seizure, and afterward, you can talk perfectly to yourself but not to others for a few hours, sometimes until you fully come around.

If it was a very bad grand mal seizure, it could be one to three days or even a week before you get back to yourself, or sometimes having a few in a day can be like the feeling of someone who has been out drinking alcohol straight for a week.

The best thing to do if you ever see someone having a seizure is to just massage their throat so they won't swallow their tongue and lay them on their side, putting something under their head like a cushion and letting the seizure pass. Then, just let them come around. If it's not over after five minutes, then call emergency

Epilepsy is something that can destroy you if you choose to leave it like any other condition such as greed, looking perfect, and so on. One of the main things that bothered me the most was having to take all the medication, even the ones that didn't work at all. The side effects had a repetitive routine.

First, it's just me wondering which step in life will be next like searching for enlightenment or something, never realizing at the time that this alone might be a step towards achieving that goal in the first place. Then I start blaming myself for what I have and telling myself to cope with it and get a life because thinking like that is a waste of energy and time. And, at times, that irritating voice would keep coming back up, telling me I'm nothing and so on. But this was also a perfect tool to toughen me up. Then there would be depression, followed by suicidal thoughts from feeling self-destructive.

Also, if someone sees someone having a seizure, you never put your fingers or anything else near their mouth. Their strength can be up to ten times more than normal and the jaw is the strongest muscle in the body. I took everything to heart when I got a little older and worried about all the small things like wondering what people think of me when they see me having these seizures. I mean, I was a nervous wreck anyway. The ignorance of people had just caught up to me many times. I was also in a place where I was not so sure about what I wanted to do with life or will be allowed to do rather than being able to do, I should say. The more you feel the ignorance of people, I feel, the more you become self-destructive. Then you are drained or tired and start taking things to heart and this is a big thing.

Why should I have bothered with what people thought of me in the first place? My head was in overdrive for years. I had no interest in anything except trying to escape from faults I saw in others rather than having them see the faults in me that were a lot more viewable to the physical eye. I knew if I ever started drinking, I would not have much longer to live or would not have been as loyal to myself to be able to continue fighting rather than give up on myself. So I never touched alcohol because as I was depressed and wanted to escape, my life would have been ruined and that position would have made life a lot more difficult.

But I did start drinking on my twenty-second birthday, as the depression was finally gone by then. Funny enough, the alcohol managed to calm me a little and the number of seizures I was getting back then. But I guess the reason for that is that epilepsy has something to do with your nerves and after drinking, you couldn't care less about anything as you're not aware of what you are doing anyway.

I also traveled around Ireland every weekend on my own as I was always the explorer and could never handle being stuck in the same place with the same daily and weekly routines all the time.

So, each week after work, instead of getting drunk and wrecking my insides later on in life, which is how I saw our Irish culture behave by choice while I was given a separate condition to face, I preferred to go to different places. I wanted to see what other people were like and see if I could link the difference in counties around the country to the difference in cultures in cities around the world that I would visit later in life. I'd just pick a county and get the bus there from Cork every Friday after work.

It was great fun knowing that though I was restricted from doing these kinds of things in a car of my own because of what I had, I was doing them anyway just like people take a year out of work and go traveling after college before they start a career.

This gives you a taste of freedom and satisfaction by just living in the here and now — like a rebel, which is also the nickname for Cork people — when you have every right to live like that.

I was full of energy and spent most of my time outside alone. Even when I started making friends, I just preferred to be alone, having to answer no one and having no plans. In primary school, it went well with no people mocking me. However, in secondary school, it was a different story as I was being mocked every day. Some people in the class even pre-tended to have seizures and laughed at me having one, which I would see when I was just coming out of one. But I was having none of it, which was what caused me big problems in secondary school, which I will explain more in detail in the chapter about the education system.

I had to fight off half the class mocking me and ended up fighting one of them every day. I didn't care how long they were going to be causing trouble or how big and tough they were, but I didn't let myself go down without any dignity. In the end, I had to leave school as I found it hard to learn and hard to even want to learn too. I used to see years ahead anyway and wondered if what I was learning there would be relevant later in life. I also saw how my parents had finished school and college a long time ago and had to struggle with some things in life. This made me question how important this was, and the seizures got worse. I went from having one a week to two a week or about six to eight per month.

At that time, I was fifteen, and we lived in a pub out in the countryside, so I came up with an idea after leaving school to wash cars for people when they came into the pub for a drink. I made good money out of it from the loyal customers. Then, a year later, I got a bicycle and started cycling to people's houses and washing their cars and windows for them.

I just had to make something out of my life no matter how difficult it was or how old I was. Staying at home waiting for the next seizure to happen while feeling self-pity and self-doubt felt much more difficult and insulting to me.

I can't say I was worthless, but I felt that everything I wanted to do and was well able to do, was not allowed because of epilepsy. So I had to simply change my tactics and do all these things in other ways, but at the end of the day, everything happens for a reason.

I think we all go through the same amount of difficulty differently throughout our lives. Some get ill and some make the wrong choices in their personal lives and don't have the energy to bring themselves back to their potential selves. Only three words made me change my attitude in living with epilepsy and start expressing myself, and those three words were: This is life!

What would your response be to such a true saying? I also got myself several jobs in the construction industry and worked hard through them all while I was still having seizures weekly. I began to struggle when I was twenty after I was put on a drug called Neurontin, which caused side effects I could never forget. They were the worst ones ever, and twenty times worse than having any seizure as well, and a lot more constant. I slept whenever I could rest, and the mood swings were unpredictable as to if I were bipolar. I might be in a good mood one minute and lose my temper the next for absolutely no reason. These were the routine effects this drug caused.

I went into a deep depression shortly afterward, as if I had given up on life completely. I stopped talking to everyone. I was letting myself go downhill rapidly as if I only had a few weeks to live, which was not how fast I gave in normally.

A few months later, I was put on anti-depressants. Taking anti-depressants for what another drug caused makes no sense anyway, and the doctors wanted to put the dose of both the Neurontin and anti-depressants up. But I didn't feel much of a difference, so I just said to myself: I can't depend on these to do all the work for me, I'm myself and it's up to me to solve my problems, not the drugs. So I threw the anti-depressants away and felt great for a short period and stopped taking them.

But a week later, I felt terrible as if I had hit a brick wall and was close to a nervous breakdown. I knew this was a re-lapse from all the chemicals leaving my body and it was only temporary but I still would not take them. I felt a bit better knowing that I can prove to myself that I can find a way of fighting through depression without being medicated again.

I'm one of the stubborn types who do not want to learn and read anything about whatever problem they have is having it takes up enough time of their lives wanting to know everything about it, and they start getting caught up in that, adding more difficulty to their situations just because they read about it somewhere.

So it's better to solve one issue at a time rather than know so much and solve so much at a time. When you already know too much about it, you will only start confusing yourself with an overactive imagination.

I looked up the side effects of Neurontin, since it was the only drug that pushed me to my limits, and one of them was unexplained death! It should have just said suicide since it was well able to make me feel that way!

A few months after taking it, I was looking forward to ending my life on this drug in a place I felt calm. Yet, I was not aware of the people it could, and would, affect and what the point was of coming this far in life. Also, ending it suddenly now did not make enough sense for me to go that far. I never thought that there would ever be a chance to see the world or learn to live and cope with such reality.

But, by saying that now, I feel like I'm being a hypocrite, and that's the difference from who I was then since my friend saved me from doing it, to who I am now. Back then, all I wanted was an end to the misery that the drugs and what I saw in society were creating, not the illness.

I was in a deep depression for a few years and completely run down. I did not even know the meaning of the word depression anymore. I didn't even know the meaning of stress. That's how slow and lost I was. I felt practically isolated from everything. My life had no structure and no meaning and I was at rock bottom. I was nothing and felt nothing but pain. You could kick me up and down the streets, insult me, abuse me, rape me, stab me☐and it wouldn't have made me feel any worse because I was already, in my mind, just a piece of filth praying not to wake up the next morning or to have cancer instead of side effects. I was gasping to escape the way I felt and the atmosphere I lived in. My spirit was dead. So, in a way, I was dead but still breathing.

I often thought of taking an overdose, but I thought to myself, That's too easy. I need something that involves pain because it's all I can feel. People say suicide is a selfish thing to do, but they haven't got a clue how it feels. So that's a little like someone saying love is a beautiful experience from someone who has never been in that type of love.

It's not as if you wake up one morning not feeling great for a while and start thinking, Now life's been pretty shit and there is not a lot going on for me at this point, so think I'll end my life even though I'm not sure where I will go or I'm not aware I was given a life to experience and live through.

You don't have a clear head wondering how your friends and family will feel. You're on a total overdrive on a different level altogether, where nothing makes sense and there's no hope and you can't see any way forward. It's a total black hole like hell that some find impossible to get out of as if you keep climbing yet the stones keep falling on you and you keep running out of breath.

It's kind of like someone who spends forty to fifty years of their life in jail, comes out to a different environment, not knowing where to start or how to live like a normal citizen. So they either start getting into trouble again, isolate themselves from everything or have a total breakdown. Feeling confused and overwhelmed and relapses because they are not sure how to take the first step forward.

They cannot be blamed. Nor is it their family or friends who should be blamed. It's not their fault that they cannot see anything good in life or are so far behind in the system than they expected earlier in life. The rest of us, who are not getting any support, find themselves worthless and not needed. They're dead inside with a head like a time bomb and can only think of ending their lives if they can't achieve what they feel they have to. They hate who they have become and do not feel loved because they don't love themselves.

When you're that far down with no one to understand you, you stop living and become more of a zombie than a human. Success at this level is to try and find happiness and explore who you are.

People can argue repeatedly about this, but at the end of the day, this is the real side of it, as I was that way for almost a decade. My biggest argument over the way we treat each other is that this is all done with our mouths. We say such harsh things about each other with such rage and anger. Our human nature causes so much trouble and long-lasting pain from our frustrations. We bitch to each other as if we run on fuel. We need to look at one another and see positive things in each other, not put each other down all the time and be jealous of one another, because we are all equal at the end of the day, with separate meanings to life and separate journeys.

Everyone on this planet is going to die one day and it's the only thing all of us have to do. That's a fact. Your lives, your property and you only have to die☐the rest is experience.

So why make your lives so miserable and put a drive on making things more difficult for yourself? Respect one another and stop trying to be number one all the time, because that never lasts. Those things are always going to be temporary.

We're all gifted with something. We all have different needs, and, most of all, we're all the same species on the same planet for one life. I do think that everyone's life would be so boring and numb without having one big issue that always makes them feel insecure. And what are people's biggest worries? The people themselves. They would not have the drive to succeed. I mean, if you have no problems, you have a little conversation with anyone else who does. When I say numb, I mean left out and bored. As people who suffer depression or overcame it would understand life's meaning quite well; experiences are personal facts to self-discovery.

Temporal lobe epilepsy

Epilepsy was a difficult enough neurological brain disorder to live with when ignorance played a very large part against it. After all, look at the word 'ignorance' for instance, where the people with it were not fully accepted into the society and more were seen as a disappointment in some aspects, depending on how bad their condition is or was, just like any other particular disorder or conclusive ongoing situation.

Epilepsy is also known as the 'sacred disease'. You could say the manipulation the medications can cause inside the body of the person was another illness in itself. Because the inside would equal the level of ignorance and hardships people had on the outside except for the inside of a person can-not really be seen or explained, and, if it could, would be seen or understood as genocide.

Then there is the fact that there is not a lot of satisfying research exhibited to show what exactly causes it in the first place, or many other disorders, and how they all began to grow so quickly, with various types worldwide. They have proceeded to be the center of people's life problems, dictating how they live, depending on their character too, of course.

It has been set to prevent sufferers from manufacturing a different style of life. Why would many be driven, when they are not accepted in the first place unless they ignore the arrogance against them and give the finger to society, just like elites and corporations can do to countries?

Same as why should a poor person live the lifestyle of a rich person when some would rather be ignorant about what the rich have, and go on to pity themselves about what little they have themselves. And behind closed doors, they could be better off in other ways and have a better marriage or better health or better neutral lives due to taking fewer big risks in life, but they would still decide to be ignorant as a mechanism to fit some way into the rich person's lifestyle.

Events such as head injuries, and close links to autism-like Asperger's syndrome, are instances where epilepsy can begin to appear. Even simple things, like ongoing chronic stress, can precede it as many people start getting it at certain stressful times of their lives. But, as I said earlier, people can survive having the illness itself, without any hesitation, if the ignorance from the lack of knowledge people have about it was eliminated through educating them, just like childcare has become a subject people are being educated about.

And interest should be established in people's concern about it with more respect and open-mindedness, so that cures can be found quicker and people stop getting sick. More people will become educated this way, rather than worried or frustrated.

Depending on how bad people suffer from it, it is usually a matter of principle to be yourself at all times. This goes for anyone with any challenge, which may intervene in why I was never that interested in fitting into society so much — not that I had anything against society or people doing whatever floated their boat, but I was more concerned with what society was all about, as I never saw a need for civilization when community spirit completely overpowers it in the first place.

There is more meaning in any community compared to society. I was always looking at bigger pictures than what was actually going on around me — sort of like a journalist in some ways, but in other ways, I would rather watch than be a part of it myself. If I saw it as a good thing, I would get involved; if not, I would stay well away.

So, in some aspects, or better still, I was a lost thought in a monitored world, as if I was in another dimension looking in from the outside. When I was growing up with it, not a lot of people knew so much about it, and I remember at one point people thought they would catch it off me if they touched me and called it a disease rather than an illness or disability.

From the very start, I felt ignorance enormously. The name Electric Eddie often appeared, and it was just something I got used to whatever the case. I didn't know how to express what it was like to live with it back then. I had it and was in the atmosphere of learning to deal with it, so I didn't have a choice but to deal with it. The people creating this ignorant atmosphere around me, pitying me, were the people who were creating something harder for me to deal with than the illness itself was creating.

If there was an actual law put against ignorance, I'd say the world would be at peace, since there is a law pretty much against every other behavior. We would have come to terms to live in a well-mannered situation and an equal society where everyone could be a part of something rather than trying to be ahead of each other.

The fact is, whatever your mind appears in is whatever you're surrounded with most of the time. At that time, I never understood that there were so many other types of disorders and diseases. I thought and felt like I was an outcast who was thought to wonder about things and made to suffer but for what reasons, I did not know at this time.

So, my mind began to work in a skeptic phase from a very young age, where I should have just been enjoying myself or doing whatever kids do, which I did to a point anyway. But I was always back to wondering, thinking about everything too because of the emotions I was experiencing, and reality already existed in my life. I could see that whenever someone was stressed or had a below-average attitude, I could link to their concern then, which explains how emotions are learned a lot quicker than thought and remembered as though they felt the same as music vibrates. This is just like when pain is felt from a nerve, and depression begins from ignorance in many aspects.

So you have to use your character's emotions to stabilize your concern, where the more sensitive you are, the faster you will feel and vice versa. From what I heard about how epileptic people were treated in previous lifetimes before I came along, I was so glad I did not have to be put through that. My dad said to me, one day after a few drinks out, that before it was discovered, people who had developed the condition were mistreated like second and third-class people. They were seen as prisoners and put into mental institutes because it was believed the seizures were being caused by Satan, or the devil, as we know him. It was thought that he has cast a spell on these people to cause dis-tress, which in some ways links to how I had begun to think, but I was glad I didn't have to be put through that term of un-certainty as I would have created quite a mess.

So that alone will tell how arrogant we can get during the worst times and how strongly our minds can make us believe something that is not true. So far in today's world, one in around 150 people develop some sort of link towards epilepsy. Since there are over 200 countries in the world, if there was the same belief as before, then the devil would have cast a spell on over two countries worth of people in the world. Many say America is run by the devil, but, in reality, it is the entire financial system from America to England, which is explained later in the book.

So who are the devil worshippers? Many may only have one to ten seizures through several years and stay on medication to avoid developing the problem in the first place, not that I believe medications are the answer, because how did people manage to cope without them before and still cope with the illness? Because looking back at these people helps create a stronger character than fully relying on medications with no fear about getting off them. Do they prevent most seizures from happening, or are they just another maintenance program for people to make billions of dollars and prevent certain people with certain characteristics to fit into society rather than helping them through a process that could take years to cure?

The fact of the matter is it was when Ireland was in a depression that I began to have this problem, people believe the worst of everything and also have a lack of demand towards their needs due to the lack of interest from the cloud of depression and drama the society has helped them develop. To get what you want during these times is ten times more difficult than getting it in good times. It's about what you need now, where before it was about what you wanted.

Example: You develop epilepsy in Ireland in 1980. You are an issue to society and a shame to yourself for having it, which is how people made me feel back then anyway. You develop epilepsy in New York in 1980, the fact you have it makes you someone important when it is discovered and the situation you're living is nowhere near life-threatening. It's more of a learning process. Even Britain, for that matter, has a link with America in being a step ahead in having the facilities, knowledge, and understanding rather than creating the problem, like it was known for before, for many generations.

As long as Ireland holds on to its history, rather than looking towards a future, and as long as the rich are allowed to make bigger mistakes than the middle or poor class and still maintain the lifestyle they had with most of the country paying for their big mistakes, it will only create more stress from the society's tormenting belief that everything they hear off the radio and television is one hundred percent true. This can also create toxic negative behavior.

Realistically, the media is only creating illusions of belief, instead of portraying accurate facts about how to create a culture, affecting the country's standards of living and inhibiting future developments. Media are agencies to make money out of anything dramatic that's happening. It's not about telling the truth. In some ways, they could relate to how the elderly are treated, who are the outcasts of the country and would do anything to fit back into society and not live in silence or loneliness.

After so many experiences and developed wisdom, I had seizures up until the age of twenty-three. Living with it until the age of thirteen was fine, but my biggest problem was having people worry about me and not letting me live a life when I was already on a mission, having what I had. So I had the opportunity to prove myself.

I had so many ideas and was ambitious, but this always got in the way of allowing me to fully do what I wanted, and the more I tried to accomplish anything, the further I got thrown back, all because I had this challenge called epilepsy and was always pitying myself.

And in Ireland, the culture was still so strong and people never looked overseas for anything. My life was at a complete standstill for now, as Ireland had nothing to offer to someone like me, at the time, due to what I had, except torment or sympathy.

But, being honest about it, I never saw the big picture that everyone was putting up with this big depression around them, because my mind itself had gone into depression and I had forgotten about people I knew or met, things I didn't like and places I traveled were long gone from my mind.

I just couldn't see the world as a fair society and wondered why people even bothered having kids when it's full of these situations and effects. I suppose, in another way, you could say for every time I changed my tactics, another type of consciousness and awareness developed. This was sometimes good and positive, sometimes bad and negative, both work with each other and need each other, just like males and females of a species do. I'd also like to state that this book will probably get more attention than my medical history, even though my medical history from having this condition is over 600 pages long - around three times as many pages as an average book.

I would also like to state that this book is just a book telling my story and experiences and yet I get more credit for writing this than I do for building up my medical data over 35 years which is over 600 pages long. Around 3 times longer than an average book and proves the true genocide happening for decades through the medical cartel worldwide.

Seizures in total up to 23 years roughly 3000 from epilepsy 40 grand mal seizures in 7 years from organ failure in the kidneys which were unaware of when I had it.

The name of the virus which was caused by too many medications for too long was PYELONEPHRITIS which was 7 years long that caused the organ failure and was reversed and I slowly recovered once treated and came off most medications was told to stay on for life for epilepsy.

Since then, I have been healthier than ever before.

Experience with modern medicine

I, more or less, had spent my whole childhood on medications, since I began to develop permanent epilepsy at the age of four. But I had no idea that I would have so many ups and downs, till I was nearly thirty years of age, even though I had realized very early that this was a system that was completely corrupt from the very top-down, by the people who funded it, such as elites and the oil industry, who wanted more profit for themselves rather than provide healthcare to people who are sick. 'Cause if everyone was healthy, it would be put out of business, and if it was an industry to help cure people, it should start from the bottom up in Third World countries, where kids starve to death, and so on.

You'll understand in this chapter that 'if you're sick, it's your own problem' and that the industry will find some way of making money off you or label you with some sort of condition, because, in this world, sickness is its source of revenue. So, before I start, I want to describe how to understand the behavior of this industry.

Imagine yourself being broke and your car tax is due and you don't have the funds to pay for it right now.

You are caught and brought to court, you still don't have the funds, but your car is impounded and you now have no transport. So you have to find a way to afford to get your car back first and then go to court and pay another fine for getting caught and then pay the backlog of your car tax too□otherwise, your car gets crushed.

So try and see the same thing here with the way the pharmaceutical industry is treating the sick. You're sick, and you can't live up to its standards, so you're not much use to it, so it isn't going to medicate you with chemically imbalanced treatments that will give you unpleasant side effects and make you suffer a lot worse than whatever you already have, as you shouldn't be sick in the first place. If it does some damage in the long run, and you've paid enough maintenance to suffer the consequences, then it might, one day, leave you alone after several years. This is how it works.

Or in a woman's view, this would be the best way to look at it. Imagine yourself as a single mother who has no income and the state refuses to help you financially and provide you with a place to live but has no problem making sure your child is vaccinated with around thirty-five vaccinations. Yet, you have no idea what ingredients are in these vaccinations, and just accept if your child gets any illness or disorder in the long run.

If they couldn't provide a home for you in the first place, why would they care if your child's healthy or not? The same goes for women, in today's developed world, who have trouble getting pregnant and are becoming mothers much later than twenty or thirty years ago, mainly due to the cost of living in the developed world. Which, when you look at it globally, sounds like a depopulation plan and is working perfectly. And if they do have trouble after waiting till later in life to start a family, they also have to pay for whatever treatment they need to get the solution found to the problem they have, which should be natural anyway and sometimes even have to go private and even sell their homes to try and make some-thing that happens naturally.

These are the best two descriptions I can give to allow someone's ignorance to be opened to understand the manipulation that is in the pharmaceutical industry that has now become a revenue system for the sick and unhealthy, yet does not go near Third World countries because they have no money. But it's not a complete revenue system. It's just an out-of-control industry that's probably even ahead of its time with solutions but more interested in profit since it realizes so many people are unaware of its power or just don't have the time to be aware.

One thing, I can say for sure, that created several side effects was the destruction I caused myself due to what I had. So guilt is also a heavy ingredient that causes many side effects, a little bit like hardship does in a person's place in society. And another thing to keep in mind is that as soon as the problem was sorted through surgery, I was still on all the medications, but the side effects were no longer active because I was then a developed adult, and I'll explain later what happened after I went off them all.

At the very start, when I started taking medication, I was a developing child at only four years of age, which is why I think the effects were very strong and got manageable only later when I was fully developed. So imagine putting your child on illegal drugs and allowing them to take all these drugs daily. When I started to take them, from what I remember, it was like something was torturing my head, but the ignorance of people, unfortunately, got the better of me. I believed it was all in my head and I was just looking for attention.

First, why would I look for attention when I'm the kind of person who enjoys spending time out in the open and doesn't spend all his time interacting with too many people? If anything, this ignorance made me drift apart from anyone who was this way, as I was disgusted by their ignorance, like they were disgusted by my epilepsy. At the start, I used to wonder whether there was something wrong with me or was it with them. But, at the same time, I wouldn't have asked myself that question in the first place if there was nothing wrong with me.

However, if you look back at someone like a tortured art-ist who is constantly contradicting themselves because they are usually right, but in a more isolated way because the world they live in is full of lies and manipulation due to how they are trying to expose the truth ahead of their time, the isolation of their belief tortures their character.

So when I was trying to tell the effects of these medications, it was like being at battle with one of the biggest corporate empires in the world. And I was speaking from experience and everyone else was speaking from what they were programmed to think through the advertising, on which these corporations spend over twice as much as they do on research, public speaking events, jobs, careerists.

This is similar to today's world where many believe what they see on television to be true, which is why advertising works. And it's called programming when there's much more to what's going on behind the scenes that they don't want you to know and be able to think for yourself, because then their system would fail and collapse.

The medications began to completely and utterly destroy my way of thinking disturbingly, threw obstacles of mood swings towards my consciousness, and had me gather the most tormenting and irritating side effects and feelings of going insane, where the only thing keeping me from going insane was asking myself if I was going insane.

I know that I'm not insane; anyone who goes so doesn't question themselves or believe that they are insane. Since the very beginning, when I started taking them and whenever I told someone, they wouldn't listen, this led me to start distancing myself from anyone who wouldn't believe me or, on a positive note, to stay well clear from anyone ignorant about it and go my own way in life from the very start.

Doctors were considered very important people at these times, which they are, the most trusted people around in society, to be more precise. But they were not trusted by me as I already had experience from an industry that paid for their education (the pharmaceutical industry) and felt it was orchestrated by whoever funds it and knew the effects of medications very well that the doctors were giving me.

The doctors have much bigger egos than the average people in society do and are only general practitioners, not gods or saints. And it was like life was easy enough with epilepsy even though I was getting about two or three seizures per week, but now with these medications, I was being forced to take it, making it twice as hard, especially when my mother was trying to keep me on them, telling me I'd die if I stopped taking them. She would never listen to what I was trying to say about the effects of them, which was like trying to bang my head through a brick wall. I presumed I had to take them to live or that I would probably die, which is what I was being told over and over from her to keep me on them.

As a child, this is a hard decision to take from the effects they are causing. The effects were like a jackhammer going on in my head twenty-four hours a day, seven days a week, similar to being hung over from alcohol, when you become self-destructive and start blaming yourself that you're nothing, you're just a waste of time and that nobody will ever want anything to do with a waste of space like you. You think you're a disease who's going to live in isolation and that this is good enough for you.

Try and imagine that level of torment going on over and over from chemical effects that you can't explain how your mood swings into episodes of emotions, mostly giving in to your lower self that is, which is how the sick people are conditioned down with neglect being self-destructive because they have what they have in the first place and it's their fault.

I remember the first time I met my local G.P. (General Practitioner), Doctor O'Brien, in Cork in a very small waiting room, which is now a taxi base; he looked respectable and intelligent and was very approachable. From the very beginning, I wondered why he was being so nice as I was conditioned to the abuse that the medications were causing at this stage or, should I say, was still trying to battle their effects.

So I was not very civilized to him at all as I wondered if his occupation had any link at all to this industry that he could be just as fooled, despite being educated, as others were with ignorance. Even though I was only a child, I started to be able to learn the system from the suffering I was going through like the saying is no pain no gain.

I was still able to think logically from a very young age but was incredibly disturbed by the side effects the drugs were causing. As I was explaining the effects to the doctor more and more through the years, all he was able to do was put me on other medications and off others to see how that goes and work with the other doctors in Cork Medical Centre to try and find a solution, so, to a degree, I became more self-destructive with this industry and more skeptical, wondering if doctors like him know what they're doing or, should I say, know what some of the medications they give can do. Because he is still a doctor and should know about what dam-age some medications can do or at least the statistics of them without been ghost-written. This would, unfortunately, be seen as negative thinking because of the jobs it creates and hopes people build from it, which is understanding because, without medications, many people in his position could be without a job.

But now that I'm grown up, I see he was a good doctor regardless and has helped many other people too. I was only one of his patients, normally his solutions were just to ease me off one medication and on to another, sort of like someone keeps putting oil into a car but never really realizes to change the type of oil and fully service the car to fix the problem.

I later wondered who was funding all these medications and was not able to come up with any cures, and there was no research I could find to answer any of the questions I had that would finally put my mind to some bit of ease. At this stage, the internet was not even out, never mind the realization of an industry being behind the whole system or whoever funds that industry in the power of the whole system, which from my research is the Rockefeller Foundation.

This is a bit like people in Europe who just go along with the EU project but never ask who is funding it and are in control of it all from the start. The side effects from the medications I felt were like complete genocide as if they were trying to kill me, and I wondered if someone was trying to kill me and others by medications. It was the only thing I could feel that would answer all the manipulating emotional abuse these medications caused inside me, and to those in the physical world who don't feel it, it showed someone who's sick and being treated with better medications than before now so they're stuck in a bubble thinking all is well now and they're getting somewhere.

That was the difference between what you see and what you feel, like the external world we see but the internal world we feel in us and just know from gut instinct. I didn't think the people who provided them were able to understand either, such as pharmacists since they're just in the big system and don't understand it. Were they there to help the sick or to prof-it from them?

The culture was at this point that the pharmaceutical industry was there to help and it had one hundred percent trust; however much it makes and however many jobs it creates, its goal was still to help the sick, even though it makes more in developed countries. People in Third World countries get better faster and it spends more on advertising and marketing than research.

So I, as one of their profitable patients, had learned shortly that they are not there to help but only consume and profit however bad your suffering is, and the truth is always going to come out in the end when the big bubble bursts. My instincts told me from the beginning that this was a scam but not a one hundred percent scam. And the longer I took medications, the more my mind was saturated with poisoning thoughts that were scattering disillusioned views and stopping my mind from being able to learn properly along with everyone else in school. Nothing ever made sense to me because I was learning from the heart from this reality experience I was living with and by feeling the reality of what was happening, rather than by memory or by the left brain conditioning like the system teaches us to be trained and programmed.

So I viewed ways of creating other systems of what life's really about, and school was just a myth in my eyes like indoctrination to just survive. As I used to say if we're all not compatible, then why are we all learning the same system? And I began to fight the pharmaceutical industry that was only there to profit off the problem that I couldn't control. No one understood except me from a gut feeling, so the issue goes on. It made me wonder whether the doctors knew what they were talking about every time I went for a check-up, because the more I went, the more pills were being prescribed. And I used to question myself how people used to live without pills. Like the Romans and Greeks and so on, what happened to all of them who had any illnesses? And how many people are making a living out of actually helping the sick now rather than curing them? I would never dream of earning money from working with the sick! Getting by, yes, but big wages, God no, I'd rather die because if that's how someone thinks then the last person they will be able to live with is themselves because it's themselves they will have to answer to.

Things like this used to send failure in the back of my mind in that department, and the more I was disrespected for explaining what these drugs were doing to my mind, the more I became an issue to fit in with anyone as it was in some ways too hard to believe the irrational thoughts and feeling I used to explain and I was seen as an attention seeker. Yes, I was young, yes, I was bold, but I was not letting chemicals manipulate my way of thinking when others were on my back telling me how to cope with epilepsy, which was not the problem. It was just a vicious circle that never came to a standstill.

I always presumed whoever was running this industry were highly educated and knew exactly what medications can do and viewing that equals delusion for society as God wouldn't ever allow something like that, even though it happened in Nazi Germany already, and history always tends to have a way of repeating itself when ignorance is a economies' revenue system.

But then as the years went by, more and more people were developing illnesses that were never around and became sicker and went to the doctors for the cause of it when they were literally put on medications and not exactly told what's wrong with them.

I managed to view the real world from a very young age and began looking at rich countries and wondered if more and more are apparently getting sick there and then wondered whether poor countries catch all these new illnesses too and what happens to them since they don't have money. These were the things that never made sense to me. It's like a feeling that can tell you the truth, such as love, and when it's learned, it never goes as for a memory it comes and goes and thought has to be studied.

The top ten pharmaceutical companies today have a re-search margin that equals up to 165 countries'

G.D.P. (Gross Domestic Product). They've been overmedicating people and engineered societies worldwide for several years, I believe. Over one hundred thousand Americans are killed by prescription drugs each year only in American hospitals, which is over half of the UK population that is prescribed drugs. Over half a million in Ireland are on pills for anxiety and depression alone which equals the population of County Cork, where I'm from.

If those deaths happened in another country in that small period of one year, World War would break out, even though war is waged at home by spreading dynamic fluids into their bodies that are shutting down parts of their system bit by bit to put them on more medications and make more profit from their so-called disability is acceptable. Ireland's culture was still very strong when I began taking medications and everyone believed that these medications were only there to help me, as medications were always the answer. I knew point-blank they were not all good for me. I even began to think they were going to kill me if I don't find a way out of this but was made to take them and suffered the consequences year after year and couldn't hide the fact of not taking them.

During my childhood, I spent most of it being hyper at the beginning and did what any other kid would do and didn't feel bad but knew my mind was changing rap-idly month after month, year after year with thoughts of how systems are created in this country to this world for people with problems. I was so scared to death of ever going into a mental hospital later in my life as I did not know my rights other than as a citizen.

I would sometimes cry from the thought of it when I saw the state of them on the telly and hoped I would never have to face going to one because one way or another, I thought I would never get out of there if I was ever put in. I knew they would come up with new evidence and create a bigger problem, fearing at the same time that somehow I would probably be put in there, thus this fear began very early in life. And I tried to stay good but still didn't put up with anyone's arrogance bullying me out of their frustration, seeing me as a bigger problem than I could have been. I began putting up a wall I had at this point for nobody to dare feed off what I was facing in the future.

During my teens, my behavior was increasingly ranked as temperamental as I was going through the usual stage of hormonal changes and the medications I was taking were also doing their thing□messing around with my system of thoughts and feeling that nobody at all could understand unless they experienced it themselves. This was quite understanding at this point and it made me feel increasingly more impatient. I began to wonder was someone trying to kill me off with the medications and have others think they're there to make you better because when you look at a medication's side effects, you find there are numerous other medications out there for each side effect alone, so how can it make sense these things are for the better?

It would be like someone betting 20 dollars or euros to win back one, how does that make any sense? The power the industry had over patients, I felt, was unbelievable. Anyone would listen to the doctor before the patient because the patient is sick, which is understandable. They don't know anything about the doctor's education and know things like they may be educated with funding from the shareholders of the higher industry like the pharmaceutical, even though they're on quite a comfortable wage from the state that makes money from doing business with these massive corporations. So to me, I like to call doctors health bankers, who are caught in the big monopolized system that think they are doing good.

I was the one apparently with the problem in my body twenty-four hours a day, seven days a week, but was never taken seriously, and it made me feel like a manipulating cost-ing failure over and over as my views of the way the manipulative world of power structure was completely blinded, though I don't blame anyone. I blame people's belief in professionals, thinking they're only there to help and are always right due to their knowledge. Is that why we have only one percent of people owning the wealth of most of the world then? Who taught them their practice? The pharmaceutical corporations! Who funds the education in universities that they learn?

Pharmaceutical corporations! Who's behind this corrupt industry? Whoever the shareholders of it are, like the Rockefellers!

A perfect example is as soon as World War II finished after the great depression, another world of the industrial revolution began, and people began to get caught up in themselves, thinking of qualifications and all these extra career choices and colleges. Identities were appearing everywhere once qualified, and people who were qualified were inflated and believed they were professionals when they were only consumers.

This process of us believing we know everything in our qualification, once we are certified, makes us more ignorant than we realize into the left brain slavery system. It's a simple saying, you know, how to do whatever you were thought, but it doesn't say to allow your ego to get the better of you once you suddenly start to work in the real world. And today, over 1 trillion of America's debt is from college debts.

And some of the people who've been living in the real world are known as losers and don't have a life of hopes or anything demanding just because they might choose not to live in the material world as much as others. I've always asked myself who taught these doctors everything? And who came up with how to run all these systems and mental institutes in the first place? Doctors, nurses? Were they people who had lost their mental health at one stage or are they just trained to work in that environment that's funded by the pharmaceutical industry, which itself is funded by the oil industry which many countries go to war for? Until I realized, it was all the pharmaceutical industry-funded by very powerful, elite, psychotic people who should have been the top patients in it for very long periods and sanctioned along with it.

And who comes up with laws that everyone's now breaking day after day like using mobile phones while driving, drunk driving, which has been around for centuries, along with speeding? Why build cars to go faster than the speed limit then, or serve more drinks in a bar than you're allowed to have while driving C.B.S. speakers that lorry drivers used before mobile phones and never had any laws where you could not talk on them while driving. In other words, I guess you could say new laws coming out in today's world contradict old ways of behaving as if we are being programmed to almost behave like robots.

And medications are a perfect match to make some people believe they are sicker than they are and create some illness for them to give them some place of identity, especially in the elderly who have the most money and feel tired and isolated. And the more people who allow something to be wrong with them, the more a society builds up demand for these pharmaceutical psychopathic corporations because we all want to be in the same union. When we're not, we start playing comparison with each other to regulate the self-destruction and self-inflation we act.

I know I had epilepsy, which is grand, but then in my teens, from the behavior I was experiencing, all this belief came up that I may also have Asperger's syndrome, which played more drama in my life. When my local doctor was con-fronted about whether he thought I had Asperger's too, which can be linked to epilepsy, he shook his head and said, "No, Eddie doesn't have Asperger's!"

I knew I did not have it and wanted to start laughing at that too, but due to my family's belief that some of its characteristics may add up to how I was behaving at home, I was drawn into looking it up myself to see if it was a possibility. Some aspects of it fitted certain behaviors I had materialized but not all of them, like not looking people in the eye and being artistic.

But the fact is, I couldn't look anyone in the eye for years due to my nervous system being controlled by all these chemicals in my system and thoughts gathering around like an outside universal program. There was also the fact that when I did look anyone in the eye, it was like I could see right into their soul and tell whether they were being honest or manipulative.

So, in another way, I believed I knew more and wasn't going to listen to anyone's lectures if they were not experienced in whatever they were talking about.

I always knew it was the medications from the time I was in primary school, while I was still developing. A perfect example is a time I stood up and threw the table up in fifth class. This was the time I began acting up and had been put on another new medication. I did the same thing in secondary school due to bullying and had been put on a new medication that time as well.

I was sent to Dublin for temperament treatment, which was after secondary school, and that was another time I changed. But I cannot say it was one hundred percent medications making me act up; forty-five percent of it was the atmosphere I was living in and forty-five percent the side effects from medications while I was developing.

Dublin Psychiatric Centre was another place where I was sent to get treatment when I felt suicidal from the medications I was on. However, I was never forced to go into any of these places. So I knew quite well all these medications together were like a controlling cocktail and had disturbed how I think and operate my life. If anything, they were slowly going to kill me if I could not find a way out of the system.

So I quit them completely, after coming back from Dublin Medical Centre, without telling anyone and stayed off the whole lot for a week and felt so great about myself☐the confidence just merged back into my system. I didn't care about having epilepsy or getting seizures once I wasn't going to be forced to take them again for epilepsy. I couldn't get over the difference in my mind.

It was like a total detox and all these disturbing effects that were hard to explain were disappearing, so I had to go and tell my mum with excitement that I felt so much better after giving up on the medications. She went absolutely mad and told me to go back on them immediately, and I said, "I don't want to. They are wrecking my mind. I can't think straight from them and I feel much better now."

She said, "I don't care, you're to take them or you will be dead!" to try to scare me. That didn't scare me a bit back then, though it was too late. If anything, it made me think that if I have to go back to these kinds of side effects again and it gets worse, then all I have to do is stop taking the medicine to feel better, and if I die, so be it!

But soon after that, which was just a few hours later, a big grand mal seizure came on. My mother called an ambulance since I told her what I had done. I was on my way to the hospital in the ambulance and woke up with drips hanging off each arm along with patches on me and said to myself, I don't know what to do anymore it is an ongoing circle like fighting the tide!

The seizures were only becoming more frequent due to me going straight off them rather than putting the dose down and coming off them gently, which I would have never known or tried that young. I needed an escape from it because I was sick and tired of living this mad-circled life and wanted to be accepted into the real world for a while if it was any bit real.

I became an out-of-control freak of nature altogether, and life was not exactly a walk in the park. Every medication I had taken at this stage had a new side effect to it, and each time I went to the doctor for a check-up, every few months from the age of five to twenty, it was the same routine with the same questions. I became impatient; I was slowly being classified as insane or maybe as an A.D.H.D. patient as well☐which stands for Attention Deficit Hyper-Active Disorder☐where I was standing up for myself, knowing quite well they're not trying hard enough due to their comfortable lifestyles and super ego to break the health system down bit by bit and fix the faults in people or cure anything.

Doctors and professors, for once, should listen to the patient! There's a saying 'the customers are always right'. Well, so is the patient, as they're living in the reality of whatever the problem is, while all the medical professionals thought skills should link the solutions with people's illnesses!

A recovered patient is also simply a born teacher or has, in another way, achieved freedom within, which is like coming back from a war, except that the war was personal, making the achievement also unique.

Before the Internet came out, it was just questions after questions with the doctors with no accurate solutions to the problem. But now the Internet can give you answers without paying for them at any time. This has brought such a fast revolution to technology and humanity, which is what fairness is rather than going to a waiting room for hours and coming out finding you have something and were just put on medications for it but were not given answers regarding the exact cause of it too, where it came from or how long it could last.

I lived a life of side effects after side effects. I was miles away from this egotistical world of false illusion, which was a good thing to an extent. But what rattles my mind day after day is the tolerance of people's beliefs that were in a civilized world when things like this are going on to justify the world's population and create more revenue from the sick and the elderly.

Greed is considered a success today, while ignorance is the characteristic that allows it but is never full or fulfilled. This is why it continues over and over to inflate. Giving is seen as a weakness to some people, especially those who are inflating. But it heals the soul and allows the person to be a good person and over half the world's population live on fewer than 2 dollars a day and are more giving because they feel who they are where an inflated person feels what they have.

All I was ever told by doctors before the problem of the illness was ever found, was that they were going to put up the dosage of my medications to see if it will make any changes or put me on a different type while I stay in hospital which was normally a week or two every few years as that's all they ever were able to do up till I was around twenty.

Of course, see how things go from there with me knowing well I'm just being fed false hope with more side effects and should continue to not expect the best and find my solutions or ways to get better if possible. They could do no more besides put me up on them or take me off and put me on another. I also lived a very daring life at these times because I knew I had nothing to lose and everything to fight for and gain. Fear was never exactly a characteristic in my life when I had this. Only frustration was continuing over and over with the same solution, and it made me wonder about how people coped without these tormenting pills and whether they all needed them or was it a massive revenue marketing experiment till the people just said enough is enough. I was trying to find someone else in the same situation as me. I only did it towards the very end in the same city as me, which I will explain later.

This caused an enormous amount of worrying to my parents, probably about one hundred times worse than it was for me as I didn't have a choice but to live with it□but they, as parents, had stress from not finding the answers.

It made them look into whether I was going insane when I was trying to explain the side effects because they could never believe that doctors can make such mistakes. They forgot that they are educated by the pharmaceutical industry or mass medications that would fail someone's system bit by bit and have them rewire their thoughts, accompanied by fears of isolation due to lack of knowledge and belief.

These were set to break me down due to not agreeing with my system because every single human is also a corporation. Like every corporation has incredible power and corruption, so can every human. The fact the economy was in depression when the illness began when I was young made the belief I was being helped understandable. However, the truth was they never helped me at all. I just didn't have the attitude to say to the doctors that you're not putting the dose up this time, as the older I got, the more I felt I was been prescribed.

But it started to feel that maybe this was meant to be the way things were meant to be for some higher purpose, but I always wanted to know what is still causing me to have these seizures. I wanted to ask that, "All you can seem to do is raise the dose every time I come in here. So why should I take them at all? Would you doctors give them all to your kids?"

Since it has failed numerous times already year after year, it is not worth coming up here every few months waiting for a few hours, and repeating the same process. Through the years, the rage in me became stronger and stronger with anger and stress issues to follow.

But, mainly, the more isolated I allowed myself to become from the few people who were understanding, the worse I got. Every time I went up for a check-up, I got blood tests. I never knew what they were for. That, of course, messed with my head. I was never fully level-headed with myself. I normally felt mixed measures because new side effects would start like a bipolar effect each time I was on a different dose or coming off them.

I was more or less relapsing over and over. The kind of side effect most of them would cause was insomnia, which created an overactive imagination from not sleeping. All I could do was think around in circles, symptoms such as dizziness as if I was completely wired from caffeine or alcohol, seeing doubles, irritating itchiness, tiredness, and depression and manic depression, along with feeling suicidal, were always towards the end. This was an ongoing circle daily in my late teens while I was on about 16 pills a day for epilepsy with four different types of them.

That was more or less my normal daily routine on how I felt in a scattered, divided, isolated environment where I could not see myself belong anywhere to part of its criteria. I needed a kick-start to help me out of this downturn of mood swings and draining sensations. I said, "This can't be good for me. How the hell am I expected to behave properly with all these medicines that can cause multiple effects?"

Anyway, I was once put on a drug that I will never forget. It is today being sued for off-label marketing and has killed many people worldwide. I hope many other people stopped taking it. When I was on it, I tried to throw myself off a cliff. It was only for my friend Nigel who caught me in time about a kilometer before I reached the destination. I knew him since childhood. He is a protestant while I am a catholic, which shows both can get on perfectly well in this story, when before they used to kill and destroy one another. Yet, to this day, he had pretty much saved me from ending my own life.

I was on Neurontin at that time; it was an absolute silent killer of a drug. I felt like a drug addict on it who was at least seventy years of age when I was only twenty. I used to be completely fine one minute and five minutes later, I would lose my temper with a complete rage. Then I would look at myself in the mirror, pull my hair out and shout, "I must be going completely insane." I was outbound with this drug and everyone seemed to think I was fine because I looked fine to them on the outside. However, when I was alone or was away from anyone I was with, the anger geared up again. It became an ongoing routine of off-loading and losing my temper.

I couldn't tell them as they were so sick and tired of hearing my problems at this stage that they began to believe I was making it up and couldn't stop feeling sorry for myself, which was never the case. My head was just full of chemicals that did not match how my conscious mind worked while developing. I wanted to feel like everyone else for once, try to feel some way normal, stop being judged by what's wrong with me and not expect me to act like the rest of them.

If I'm going to be fed drugs day in and day out that doesn't match my DNA (Deoxyribose-Nucleic-Acid) or my system, that's more or less my answer to the ignorant people who thought I was looking for some form of self-pity when I never wanted anything like it in reality.

My old friend Nigel who stopped me from throwing myself off the cliff after going on Neurontin couldn't believe it when I later showed him the side effects of it. "My head is destroyed from it." I told him, "And I can't think any bit straight anymore except about ending my life."

He said, "But I told you to get off it." I said, "I know but I have done that before and ended up in hospital. What am I supposed to do this time because if I tell the doctor I'm doing it they won't help me."

Today, I don't understand what I could have done because I wasn't in control of myself at all with this one. After starting that, I would have rather killed myself than end up in the hospital without even thinking about how selfish killing myself could even be or whom I would have left behind. I could not even realize that, at the time, which doesn't make sense to how I usually thought. I normally had a tactic where there must be a way if I've come this far already.

Whatever way you look at it, things were not looking up once I started taking this drug, which is why he caught me by the arm and started pulling me back slowly while listening to me when I was on my way to throw myself off the cliff.

I began to forget about the fact I was on my way to the top of the cliff to throw myself off it. I gradually walked back along with him. That just shows how messed up my head was from thinking too much along with insomnia and an overactive imagination along with the effects of the drugs. To this day, I don't know if I would have done it. When I came up to the cliff, I saw the beauty of Cork harbor, which always melted me and healed any pain inside.

It was certainly no mistake that I bumped into him that time and I always tell him that he saved my life that day. Someone must have been looking over me like my grandfather or someone who I usually felt connected to in any way even though I never knew him personally.

A few weeks later, I went for a check-up in CoCork Medi-cal Centre. As usual, Dr. O' Donohue wanted to put the dose of this drug up. I said out loud, "No way, that's the last straw. I'm lucky to still be alive after taking that and, if anything, I want to be taken off it. I don't even know if trying something else is a good idea anymore. I'll nearly try cocaine or heroin rather than stay on that!"

I've been on everything else and he paused for a moment and said, "Well, there is a new one that just came out. We might be able to offer it to you while we could take you off Neurontin since it did not agree with you either." He was looking into my files studying all the medications I was previously on while saying all this. I replied, "No problem at all, belt away, just get me off this one please before it kills me."

He had a kind of stunned look on him as if he was surprised at the effect it had put on me. So, off I went back home and was told I will be given a call whenever there is a possibility of getting ahead to get medications changed over which can be a slow process. So, I started taking the new drug a few weeks later before coming off the old drug, which is what hospital stays were normally for.

I had a blast of seizures later on getting sick and so, falling on the floor, after I came around my father asked if I was okay. I felt fine and normal and he sat me down telling me I just had a very bad one. I said, "I'm grand, doesn't feel like I had."

He presumes it was stuff like Red Bull and Coke causing them or caffeine. In fairness, give me a break.

I didn't smoke or drink. Everyone else does, which I see and wonder what it's like and don't see them with much of a voice if they do stupid things like that after alcohol. I didn't have the energy to argue and didn't fancy giving them the satisfaction of knowing what my problem was seeing them drink and have a thrill with me, stuck stone sober thinking of a way out of this mess. Just to ease his mind fully knowing that caffeine didn't cause them, I gave it up for about two months.

Nothing changed, so I went back on it for a boost now and then. I was sick of having to prove to them what they think is not completely true, so I told them, "Bear with me and let me live a little because I'm not an animal. I'm a human and if you don't start treating me like one, I won't give you the satisfaction anymore, not letting you know what my problem is since it will be seen later as a dramatic problem broadcasted all over, which makes me feel a hell of a lot worse."

 They were way too worried about me and I felt I was being pushed away from the worrying, even though I moved out at the age of fifteen and got a place with a few friends. I didn't want to be worried about it. I just wanted to be treated normal and not be known as the one with problems and others thinking I just wanted to be the center of attention.

I just had my own belief in things from the reality I was living and my instincts are nearly always right along with intuition, which I always go with whatever the case. Anyway, this new drug I started to take was called Keppra and was the final drug I was ever put on for seizures.

Things were going fine once I started to take it and came off the Neurontin, which was a blessing to get away from and seizures began to stop. This was worrying me because I knew there was something in my head that more or less I wanted removed to complete the success of never having one again. This is all explained later in the story, so whether the new drug stopped them or not, I still wanted surgery.

It certainly made up for what distress the last drug had caused. Being on Keppra, I spent three weeks not having a seizure, which was good as normally I would have one or two a week, sometimes more sometimes fewer, so things may have seemed to look up to others and me. But, I wanted the surgery done whatever the case.

Over three weeks after starting Keppra, I began to get worse and started to get more seizures as often as before, which didn't bother me because I knew this was probably a relapse of not having them for over three weeks and what was causing them was the new mixture of Keppra. I knew I might be able to finally get cured of it, so I stayed positive because I had the vision to look at and I kept it as positive as I could that it would work even though I was never given a hundred percent guarantee that it would cure me. At least, I finally got an answer.

So, as I finally got the surgery which is all explained later in the chapter about Beaumont hospital I had a seizure straight after it. The neurologist Dr. O' Connell put the Epa-nutin up by 50 mg and said to stay on that level for the next few months. That was the last seizure I ever had. I don't even remember having it as it was before I woke up after surgery. Anyway, a few years later, I gradually began to come off the medication one by one, which I should have started a year ago. But, I was worried about what it could do to me. I wasn't worried about having a seizure because I knew it was over but was just a little worried that side effects would start to come while I was easing off them gradually. This is why it took me a little bit longer to begin to come off them.

The first one I began to come off was Lamictol because they were the longest I was on. I remember Dr. O' Connell telling me that I'll be coming off 50mg per month as that was the lowest dosage you could get them in. So, a few years after I had the surgery, that's what I did and didn't feel any effects except a little dizzy at times. It didn't bother me at all and I felt good making the move at last.

The best thing was that I began to see things more clearly and think differently. The more dosage I came off, the better I could see things. So, I came off the Lamictal fully after a year and went back to neurologist Dr. O' Connell for a prescription to come off the Epanutin since that was the second-longest one I was on and the same thing was done with that dosage. I came off them 25 mg at a time, as that was the lowest they were on. Again, I didn't feel much effects coming off them either and was done in a year, so finally, I began to come off Keppra, which was the only one I had left.

I didn't tell anyone about and I was looking forward to fully being off medications but was a little worried because the lowest these came in was 250mg and they were a morning and night tablet. I wasn't sure what to expect coming off them. I decided to break them in half and slowly come off them monthly. Each year, I came off one medication and by the time I got to the last, I was pretty nervous as the last time I tried this I ended up in hospital. Also, last time I had epilepsy and am now cured of it. In another way, I was not allowing this to dictate a routine any longer of taking medicine morning and night. Since I was a child and this was my final freedom, I was happy that it was a lot of weight off my shoulders now that I could just go anywhere without packing these or anything like that or wondering, "Will I get them if I ever moved away from Ireland."

One thing I did realize during the process of coming off them was that my mind was incredibly getting sharper, my lifestyle was healthier, my moods were calmer, my way of thinking was more describable and my health was now good in general rather than fighting for it.

It became so much better. I began to wonder, "Was I right when I thought during the years of growing up that medications were a way of killing people off in masses." I know well that the developed world has an awful problem with the world's population in general, so why would they be there to help you in the first place without some tricks up their sleeve.

However, to try and get that out there and wake people up would be literally like living an illness all over again. I did stay on the minimum of Keppra in the end at only 1000mg per day that has had no effect at all. I have now taken control of regulating myself with this industry and not to go along with its regulations where profit comes before health anymore.

This industry kills more people than wars do from the cost of doing business. People need to wake up to such a massive epidemic with prescription drug effects only killing over 100,000 American's every single year in hospitals which is just above the number of words on this whole book or the number of seconds in a whole day! Roughly 20,000 are killed from not being able to access a doctor so that's five times as many deaths in hospitals from prescription drug effects than those who die from not being able to access a doctor along with another million going bankrupt due to medical costs!

Malaria, for example, kills about one million under the age of five every year, yet psychiatry being only one chapter of this psychotic pharmaceutical industry kills 500,000 people in the Western world, with most of them being over 65 every single year. Another example is cancer that makes around two hundred billion dollars per year in America yet has no cure out for it when rockets can be flown to other planets and nukes can be launched to other countries faster than ever. I would call this the American corporate nightmare rather than a dream! Two hundred billion is about as much as Ireland's entire economy per year which has over 4.5 million people in it. If there can be corruption in a small economy like Ireland and cancer can make as much in a bigger country than smaller countries' whole economy adds up to. There should be some serious regulation on who controls and profits from such a massive psychotic system.

As of 2019, the World Health Organisation has Highlighted a World Patient safety day about this global epidemic stating that at least 5 people are killed every minute by modern medicines. And the global cost to this is 40 to 50 billion per year. Where I'm a clear example of who came out the other side of it twice.

The virus caused from detoxing from years on to many medications (Polypharmacy) lasted 7 years after but was unaware what it was and led to kidney failure causing Grand Mal seizures rough amount:

40

Almost led to being on a waiting list for A KIDNEY TRANSPLANT. Antibiotic and few dialyses and recovered.

I would also like to add I am not Anti Vaccine just because I know how corrupt these drug Companies are with

Medications, am for safe Vaccines and do Hope that the Vaccine market is not left to adopt the same Mafia Type business models as Polypharmacy has done that became a Global Epidemic.

I have got the yellow fever vaccine as an example which is for life before visiting sub-Saharan Africa, and it has had Zero effect, plus now studies have shown that updated yellow fever should also cover covid infection. At least this vaccine is almost 100 years old and has a very high safety record. So why would it allow a for-profit strategy to monopolise its safety record now?

Rich heritage to cancel culture

Here is a perfect example of how the process of families, cultures, and countries' behavior can distract anything positive from being started due to the atmosphere of their lives, cultures, or religious beliefs as well as the stress they were under or the power they had over one another. Except, this was through childhood, whereas today we all link a gap between rich and poor from the pressure we built in the society and the material work we put into wealth for ourselves rather than treating each other equally and searching within ourselves emotionally and spiritually.

Also, in some ways, this gap that was created between me and my brother was from emotion where blood is thicker than water and can never be broken whether you want it to be or not. Like the bond a child has with his/her Mum can never be fully destroyed. Fighting against it became harder later in life as hatred was starting to deteriorate because it would have otherwise destroyed me in all types of ways. Whereas the gap in society was from ignorance and tactics in economics from those in power run by their ego and superego - false self and super false self

- and on top of that, they say we are only using ten percent of our brains. If we are only using ten percent of our brains and have been orchestrated by people running from their super false selves then something is very, very wrong.

Individual people need to start taking their power back and create their systems otherwise it would come to a point where economies would be run like an ego making them false economies. Then, continents and finally the world would be run by our false selves by complete psychopaths until we got it, reversed our systems, and took the power back to us as communities on a global scale. In a way, you could say, what societies' ignorance was doing to me, governments were doing to societies and continents were doing to each other. This is due to our ignorance of needs that mean nothing in reality. Because reality in the end is your reality.

You only have one person to answer to in the end and that's yourself; no one else can take from you whatever you feel or know or share. The problem people have in general is that many are either living their lives for someone else or are too ignorant or well-off to know who they are to live in the moment to have peace of mind. It's the same as the way inflation and deflation work. You're inflating and becoming self-destructive and ignorant where pride, lust, and ego rule you. When you're inflated, you don't give a damn about the rest of the world and think the world's all great because your superego is ruling you and you don't even know it. So, why should any of these two characteristics be running the show? Why would these two have the attitude to want to help when they're both self-centered characteristics and not able to feel others' pain or what goes on in other countries and continents?

I and my older brother Gerard have never really seen eye to eye because we know exactly how to get at each other's nerves and how our minds work testing each other out like most business people such as oil tycoons, pharmaceutical shareholders, and bankers, countries like England and Ireland, America and Russia, families and so on would test each other.

We have always had a hazardous relationship in competition rather than brotherhood and tested every ability on each other. We were just as stubborn as each other to want or try to get on too but too immature to try when the damage was done. Too much immature behavior was in my character to function any system of growth for the sake of peace or surrender rather than feeling resentful from him from an early age. I also saw him as a tool to take out my stress about the fact that he was the one who crossed me in the first place way too many times and is my blood.

In the long run, all memories of tolerated sadness were never forgotten until it was time to mature from the mind of hectic circumstances and learn from the point of view that everybody subtracts needs and repairs them in other consider-ate ways to grow their character to the next level of consciousness if they can make it that far.

While some may heal, others may stay neutral and when time has measured growth of maturity, a system of enlightenment can arrive. Civilization exists; except in a person, it's not civilization: it's peace of mind, self-realization, self-acceptance. Everything between us was way too raw and it was long and drawn out to the last that it would be a final make or break before the run up to making peace with each other before we had to go our separate ways in adulthood and create our own families and knowing one another was just a myth at this point as interest as brothers were over.

But, we were still the same blood and the speed of growing up was limited with value and excelled from emotion and there was no trust to even consider having any civil relationship. There was no love in my department, which doesn't ever seem to annoy me as I got older because, in reality, a lot of families have this link issue and just manage to create an urban civil relationship like they don't know each other but know they are related like countries don't but know they are all human.

My side of the story between him and me began when I was five. At the time, I used to look up to him with him being older than me. He acted like a second father figure being the oldest. In my eyes, he was the leader of the bunch since he didn't cross me, so I used to copy everything he did and wondered what he had planned and tried to be his chief brother keeping up with him.

Despite the fact, he couldn't handle me and began to get sick of me quite quickly. It annoyed me and confused me, which had me think about how I must act around him and why. But, I had my way of doing things the more I was let down. Each time I was laughed at, I would bounce back with an idea and shortly understood the feeling of ignorance after a few of these occasions and saw that this was not a place for me to depart at all.

If this is normal, so be it. I began to drift towards a self-knowledge lifestyle thinking and imagining the country and the world as I became more evolved and thought with more perception the older I got.

I truly began to think every time I analyzed our differences that he decided to begin hating me from the start due to me having a condition that made me similar to a revenue consumer with the pharmaceutical industry.

He thought I was the problem. His alarm was to shut me out of his life and create hassle since I was already beginning on that path anyway and he was not able to deal with what I was going to be facing, which would make total sense rather than caring for me as a brother because it would be too hard to handle.

I was still standing down to nothing and always aiming high, whatever it took. Being able to make up compared to how much of a different person he was not being able to stand to any measurements without someone's help or consideration or approval. I could not remember any time where he was happy to have me as a brother except for the times his own life seemed ok or was getting better.

I felt like I was his target to push under the carpet and make sure I'll always be on a lower level than him due to his ignorance and succeed in nothing and accomplish nothing besides shame and defeat. I learned this at the start of life and it was probably the best lesson I needed to understand in the long run that we're not all the same with the same characteristics to fit into the same systems. Many of us must learn before we get a need or earn our voice in other words.

The worse thing was I had nobody I could tell this to as I didn't want to tell my parents as I wasn't the type to want to create drama or concern. I always demanded attention that I know I deserved but never wanted any drama, so all that racket going on in my mind began to build up as I never knew how to put it all into perspective and was a right hammering due to the former problems that began to manufacture between the two of us.

I was already just trying to get on with life and then this stupid pattern followed. I just couldn't get these contradictions out of my mind from being treated like dirt because of who I was and what I had and worse is why would you treat someone like that in the first place? Jealousy? Spiteful? Un-fulfilled? Boredom is what I think in the end has a lot to do with this negative behavior and desperate for enlightenment or fulfillment, same as poverty produces some people to have more ideas than the wealthy. Boredom creates some people to create more negativity due to them seeking enlightenment, as they have to seek the truth and go through all the problems to set them free.

I used to say out loud quite a lot and often even cry myself to sleep about it because of seeing that I had no friends due to what I had. It was because I have a stupid neurological condition called epilepsy even though the drugs were doing way more damage. I thought that nobody wants anything to do with me and hated everything about me. All this loneliness began to load up inside me when I was young due to the way he treated me because he is the eldest and he is meant to lead the way, not try and gain from his immature strengths to bring other people down. I began to hate him more than anything in the world as things got worse.

That day, at five years of age, I had made one close friend called Claire whom I shared most of my time with and was literally in love with the girl due to her nature. We did everything together, calling to each other every day, going out into the open fields for hours with not a bit of worry and all the rest of it.

That day she called down to me at the usual time around midnight as it was a Saturday when I was about six at this time so remember the country was just after going into severe recession too. My brother was standing up on the planks that were placed on the barrels to run up and down.

He was playing away and saw her coming close to the gateway and called me instantly, which was surprising enough as he already showed he hated my guts and said, "Eddie, tell her to just go home and not to bother coming back," with a big grin on his face as if he would get a right laugh from it□which was exactly his idea.

I couldn't see that then. All I could see is that he was talking to me, which I couldn't understand and was confused about it. So, me being stupid, I thought if I do this maybe he will let me in or just be a normal brother. So, hoping I wasn't going to be sorry for falling for his little stunts I told her where to go and she put down her head with shame, began to cry, and ran off home and my heart just dropped. I knew that was it and I would never see her again.

I still regretted it even at age twenty and have never seen her since wishing that I never did it. That was the day I began to carry guilt. I did try ringing a few times later in life and hear she is happily married today, which is great. As she ran home, I turned around and looked up at my brother and he was there standing on the barrel laughing at me shaking his head. He called me a fool, turned around, and ran off playing.

I stood there absolutely disgusted and devastated that I fell for his stupidity again with me being the sensitive person was hard enough, but I was only a kid, and he should have known better, but I guess he was only a kid too along with a bully's mind but I had the strength to deal with real life.

That was the day I could only begin to increase my hatred towards him. From then on, I wanted to make his life a living hell as the only friend I had at that time was now gone and I knew it was done and dusted due to my stupidity of listening to him to hope he will change his ways. Everything he got from there on that what he treasured I broke. I made sure I broke them: his toys and his gifts. Anything he treasured, I destroyed and I used to sleep under his bunk bed. I wasn't a great sleeper with everything on my mind and the side-effects of the medications, so I drove him mad every single night, throwing my feet up at the bottom of his bed, bouncing him up and down till he lost his temper.

I was on a mission to get back at him and make him suffer, whatever it took, for being such a bad brother who only wants to ruin me to please himself. I used to mock him, thump him and at one stage, even planned to kill him when I got older as I felt he killed a good side of me and I could not forgive his actions. My parents didn't know what went wrong with me, but I let on that I didn't know what was wrong myself because I wasn't finished with him yet, so I didn't let them know my issues with him and kept to myself, as the anger grew in me day after day.

I just let Gerard tell his side of the story, and I just nodded and said nothing, but in the back of my mind, I was far from finished with him and had already planned out my next stunt. I had become more bitter having to listen to his rubbish like he cared and was concerned about me, and he knew it too.

He seemed to know my weaknesses and strengths better than anyone else, and that's how he knew he could affect me in any way he tried. He wanted to have control over things because I never had full control of anything anyway, with the way things were even though I tried to face many dares.

Even when some of his friends would try and talk to me, I couldn't and wouldn't bond with them because I wanted nothing to do with anyone in his life as long as they thought he was a good person and especially didn't want him to know anything more about me. So from then on, I went my own way and drifted from him and everyone else in the family because I was so mad. In principle, I became a bully to anyone who was going to give me a hard time and defended myself before people like him. I gave people a bad time when they stood up to me like I was doing to him. I do regret it today, but I was young and stupid, defending myself.

A year after all this started, my mother had another child, whom I went up to see in the hospital with my aunt from the father's side, Ann. I walked into the hospital, saw my mum sitting on the chair with her green dressing gown on, and a few minutes later, they brought over Joseph which they called him in his tiny little incubator.

I couldn't believe what I saw. He was tiny and my mother said to me, "He's going to be your brother", which I was not able to fully accept due to my experiences. I just kept staring at him for a while. He looked unnatural and I made a promise to myself that day that I'll try and look after him and won't treat him the way I was being treated by my older brother. From then on, I was being a bully in school to protect myself more or less from being the first one to be hurt, as Gerard had already begun at home. Along with that, I blamed the illness for making life more difficult when it was more the medications. I just didn't want to let anyone in on the truth because I was still sad and missed my old friend Claire even though she was only down the road, whatever was there was completely dead now.

At home, I could not stand the sight of Gerard any longer, so I gradually became more of a loner and went the opposite way any time he was around. I could not stand the sight of him and becoming more annoyed by his presence every day, so I would go away for long walks in the fields, play outside away from the rest of them and just distance myself from him or whoever his with.

I didn't want to be involved with anyone close to him either due to the fact of never wanting him to know anything about me again, which is how loyal I am. So, I stayed an outsider and did my own thing like building three houses and swings and beginning to cycle. I got used to my own company, apart from a few friends I had who were not that close to me.

As Joseph grew up, we began to fight more frequently as if we were trying to get him on one of our sides and I wanted him on mine because I didn't want the older brother ruining him as well, as he tried to do it to me. Again, this was just childish behavior and wasn't exactly leading anyone anywhere, but I wasn't going to make up with Gerard in a hurry either. If anything, all I ever gave him was the anger I had towards him, and I showed him how much I disliked his character, which was completely the wrong behavior to have towards anyone in the first place anyway since I was only creating more negativity towards myself and others too.

I left things as they were then for a while and drifted further away from everyone, becoming more naive towards anyone that tried to help me in any way. Not only did I start to become more guarded but became more multi-guarded to-wards people, like I was stocking up for a war that was going to happen or something.

In reality, fifty percent of me was causing this to happen by accepting that I could, unfortunately, bump into more unpleasant people like Gerard later in life that I won't fully understand or fully be able to help to my best potential. Becoming aware of bigger possibilities and bigger corruption than what I saw or heard was a positive here. But, developing an overactive imagination and anxiety towards some major negativities was, on the other hand, a possibility that could have made me a lot more ill and unfit to live a healthy life too and could have caused a lot more self-inflicted issues without me even realizing it.

It was soon after this behavior had begun to start developing that I was being brought for my first visit to the psychologist in Cork Medical Hospital, which is where I'm going to explain everything that I experienced in this city. That chapter of my life had just started from there.

Anyway, I didn't have any problem with being sick at this stage but would use it as a tool if I was questioned about anything or wanted solid information about something I was aware of but could not find the direct truth about. With the number of things I was prohibited to do, I did them anyway just to prove a point, and other people would say that I had some behavior disorder and think about medicating me due to this behavior. I was aware that this was a possibility but I still chose to prove a point every time I was told I could not or am not supposed to do something.

Sometimes, my sister Elizabeth would try and comfort me by bonding with me, asking me, "What's the problem?"

I told her the first time that I just hated Gerard for who he was and she said hatred is a very strong word. I said, "It doesn't matter. That's how I have felt about him since I've been a child." She just threw her head to the side, gradually raising her eyes to the heavens, gave me a tap on the shoulder, and ran off playing with her friends. But because she was close to him, I knew I could only tell her so much even though she was only trying to fix whatever was broken.

So after that, I said nothing more in detail and let it go every time I had a problem and as I got older, she met a few people, as we all do, and dated them. I used to watch out for her to make sure that she was treated well by the right people, and this way returned the favor that she listened to me and wanted to know what my problems were, being a good sister. Some of them were good people, so I used to wonder if she would marry them and began to look at them as being older brothers I wished I had, that I needed for so long. But, as soon as Gerard became friendly with them, I again went my separate way and shut down any contact with them that wasn't necessary.

One day, when we lived in the public house, for example, I was out just after cleaning it, before we were opening up, and went to town to buy my first music tape, which was AC/DC. I was so happy after getting it that I went straight back home all excited about it, looking forward to showing someone before we opened the public house for business. Gerard was the first person I saw, and I showed him what I got. He looked at me with a grin on him and said, "You're sad!"

I looked up at him and said to myself, What have I done now? What is his problem with me? I just shook my head and walked away in shame.

Shortly after that, my anger grew severe every time we had a conflict. The time I smacked the other brother Patrick when he became like Gerard almost led to a bloodbath. Pat-rick, who is two years younger than me, was so angry with me for thumping him because I would not give him money when he demanded it for using his friend's computer when I asked if I could use it that he went to Gerard for support. One afternoon, Patrick wanted a fight about two weeks after I smacked him for having a go at me for not giving him money, and Gerard was up in the loft with his friends. Patrick tried to get the better of me, and I began to lose it again but this time, a lot more violently. He ran up to Gerard, and I ran like lightning after him.

Gerard said, "Stay down there", but I had gone completely mad now at this stage with rage that had never been this bad yet, and I ran up there like a monster and went for the two of them. Patrick got a big fright and caught the older brother just as I was about to smack him and ran for his life. I was up on the second floor looking down at them and they sprinted off.

The next thing I knew, I had a seizure and fell to the floor from it from being so fired up with anger. An hour later, I woke up in the sitting room. Gerard was there with the usual grin on him and said, "What do you think you were doing?" I was just waking up and he said, "Don't ever try that on me again."

Just as well that I was only coming around or I would have gone for him again. Shortly after that, he kept it up. I went for him again with a golf club when I came around and just missed his head by a few inches. I could have killed him without realizing it there and then, so I was very lucky in that way that he locked himself into the store away from me. If anything, I matured much quicker than he did, as I grew up due to my actions from my anger, stupidity, and real-life issues.

A few years after that, his twenty-first was on. I went to it and bought him a drink. He said, "You're my brother and I love you." But I couldn't open myself to hear that after never feeling it, not with all the memories and hatred I had with him. I had shut my barriers down to him a long time ago, so it was more or less an in-one-ear-and-out-the-other thing by now. Soon after that, I walked home wondering what made him say something like that, or was it due to him just having an enjoyable night with some alcohol in his system?

As I had never even drunk alcohol either at this time and didn't know what effect it can put on people's minds. I just only saw what states it puts people in, so I was analyzing why he would say that now after all these years of clashing with one another over the most stupid things.

However, I threw it to the side after a while and didn't bother thinking or putting much more interest into it. The bitterness towards him was still there inside my system. What relationship we had created and destroyed even if I could forgive him I could not forget. Nothing had changed in the long run.

All of a sudden, though, in 2000, on New Year's Eve, a breakthrough had come where we both became a little mature. This was three years later and at midnight we just made up from being tired and fed up with it. I thought that was it done and dusted. This barrier of grief is split at last, but a few days later when we were out in the pub, he was after a few drinks, I was talking to his friends and he said to them, "Never mind him. He's gay."

This began to boil my blood because I'm not and may have had a great friendship with Claire at this stage if I didn't listen to him back then. Secondly, when I was seventeen, I was nearly abused by a man who threw me down on a bed after giving me a lift and was going to drop me off in town after asking me to quickly help him bring in his suitcase and I was street smart here and knew something wasn't right and managed to escape.

I did not like what Gerard said even though he was only winding me up, having the labeled condition was on my mind too, and being the outsider of the family was on my mind.

I was back to square one analyzing why does my older brother want to shut me off and I thought I was such a big problem for him ruining his image. In secondary school as well, I was a loose cannon. Every time I broke out when someone tried to mock or get the better of me, the teachers would take me to wherever he was and leave me with him without ever realizing the relationship I and Gerard had was nothing. I saw this image on his face every time this happened that he was more or less ashamed of me showing my emotions in public and to have me, as a brother, was such a burden.

He just wanted nothing at all to do with me or could not accept the fact he had a brother who had some real issues and had no one to look up to except his parents but didn't want to tell them everything as it would only create worry, strain, and more talk.

Anyway, after all, this happened, later in 2000, my grandmother passed away in east Cork. We went to the funeral and I remember my father having a last look at where he grew up, which was always a town I liked quite a lot by the seaside. He was so proud of his parents whatever way he was brought up which was a great achievement to understand.

He was about to cry as you would while crossing the road and about to get into the car after looking at the house he grew up in for the very last time. I caught him and told him that I loved him and was proud to be named after him as he was named after his dad too who passed away when I was young. So, after that we all went to the pub, Gerard was going to Cork with a few of our cousins and I went with them.

I and Gerard talked for a while again until he was after a few drinks and wanted to go home. I wanted to go back to east Cork as I didn't see the point of going home, so he tried to tell me we're going home. I said to myself, You can't expect me to listen to you after all these years. I've been alone and said to him, "I'll go to east Cork. You can go home. I've been traveling around Ireland since I'm sixteen, so back off."

He tried to drag me over. I punched him and put him down on the ground. We were fighting on Patrick's St. in Cork City like a pair of kids. After that, he said, "You're on your own from here, boy, we're done!" And I replied to him in total rage that I've been on my own all along, so it doesn't make any difference anyway.

He went off in a taxi and I got a separate one back to East Cork. So, from then on we drifted again and stayed away from each other for a while and I grew up quickly realizing I'm going to have to cut some very serious slack here and stop this anger that is in me while I can. When I was in a real mess in the psychiatric ward in Cork Medical Centre when I was on anti-depressants and in there while I was getting the dose of them put up a few years later, my sister came and visited me, as she was always good for it anyway. For some reason, something came into my head about death this time as I was also experiencing suicidal thoughts from the anti-depressant Effexor that I was put on to up the dose of it in there.

I wondered the fact I'm here now and can't see forward at all while I'm trying to balance out all this. I wondered who would come to my funeral and that linked to me wondering if Gerard would ever visit me in a place like here? She looked at me with a kind of frown and surprise as if he had already planned to come in anyway. She said, "You would never know! I think he might want to visit you here but doesn't want to upset you as things are bad enough as it is between the two of you." I nodded and said it doesn't matter anyway. Then, I threw all that was on my mind to her as I felt my life was now over with the state I was in and told her about the abuse that nearly happened before by a guy. I added I was not affected by it as I was very low at that time of my life anyway. But, when Gerard called me gay without known anything like this I would fire up so fast and make any excuse to just lose it.

She was shocked that I kept it in for so long and said she knows some people it did happen to but least expected it to happen to me and asked if she could tell the parents. To myself, I said, "No way, God only knows how many will be told from the worry of them being told." I didn't have the energy to go into reasons for keeping it confidential for all that time, so I kind of said, "Okay, work away because I couldn't care anymore."

I wanted her to keep it quiet in a sort of "No, don't tell them" way. That evening my mum came up and was raging with me that I never told her, but I just couldn't handle people worrying about me as I felt like a total outsider with enough problems. At this stage, I didn't want to fit in with anyone anymore anyway. So she said, "I'm your mother, I do the worrying whether you like it or not," but from where I was, I couldn't consider that and never could.

 I was trying to prove points that I can do what I`m told I'm not allowed do so worrying feels like a complete burden. The next day was a little strange, as I felt twenty times better after releasing all this toxicity of information out of my system that many males can't do at all. Gerard came in to visit me, so I presumed our sister told him what I said about him. He asked how I was, and I said, "Fine how are you?" He said, "If you want anything just let me know," but again I still had my barriers shut and couldn't bond with him and said, "Don't worry about me. I'm grand."

He tried to let me know that he was there anyway. I knew it, said thanks, put up my hand, and shook his, and then he left. So, a few hours later my dad came in and was devastated with what the sister told them and said, "Eddie, you are my son, we're here to protect you and for God's sake, tell us when something happens and we will deal with it from there." I said, "Thanks, but I never realized how much I was punishing myself for situations I may have been involved in but didn't create and something like this was nothing compared to what the drugs I was on for years, which have done a lot more. Nobody took any notice of since it brings so much revenue into the economy and couldn't be able to do so much damage like I was saying all along and gave up many times talking about it."

I was drained from thinking so much, and I was in such a mess in there that I was deeply depressed from emotion, confusion, isolation, and I felt disgusted with myself and felt like no girl will ever be interested in someone like me due to what I had.

Then, I met Katie there that time, whom I did fancy a little bit. She was also a girl with very big problems. We got on good and a few days later, I was sick of being in there and signed myself out. I never went back and said my life's my responsibility to change and it's me. I must take action more and more rather than go along with the system that has not helped much. Due to this feeling, it was all just a big hoax of an industry anyway.

A few months after that, I was in the public house with James, and the depression had eased off an awful lot because I stopped putting myself down. Since I decided to sign myself out that day and took some bit of my sovereignty back, I never looked back and stopped taking the anti-depressants too which was a massive weight on me. That made me realize that whatever you decide to do is entirely up to you and you don't have to go along with a system all the time. You should never be afraid of taking back your sovereignty.

Hence, I decided to stop beating myself up all the time and try to gain more than lose so much that was given to me in ways I never allowed myself to see. When the depression eased, I began to drink a little later. I knew I would never allow myself to reach this level of depression ever again or this level of suicidal thought. On my twenty-second birthday, I drank whiskey of all drinks for the first drop of alcohol I ever had. It mellowed me out and never made me a worse person or never drank so much either.

Then one day, I was in town with James. Gerard was also there. This was the first time he had ever seen me drink and said to me, "Didn't think I'd ever been asking you this but what do you want to drink" I said to him, "A bottle of beer." That was fine and we were all talking to each other. A friend of his came in whom I knew anyway since she used to hang around with people I know.

I was talking away to her. Again, Gerard turned on me and said to her "Never mind him. He's gay again." This time I just laughed it off and didn't care what he said as I could see it was himself he was making a fool out of and was only joking too. I accepted that this was part of his character I had to accept. James just stared at him and me with a confused thought as if he didn't know what to think.

I used to think if it was Gerard who might be gay as he seemed to be obsessed with going on about gay people all the time. But, I more or less kept that on the back of my mind and said to myself, "Well, if he is, I really couldn't care because I've enough problems rather than judging someone who might be a little confused where their sexuality lies."

At the end of the day, whatever is meant to be will be. So again, we stopped talking, stopped saluting each other. A year later, just after the operation was done on my brain, which is in a later chapter on the book, I was in Cork one night and he phoned me. I missed the call but didn't call back, and he was in France when he was told the operation had been done and was a success. I have forgiven him many times but as soon as he had a few drinks in him, he would start annoying me again in front of everyone, better still make a mockery of himself I should say.

But I don't hate him anymore as I've grown up to dislike people but not hate them. That plays too many mind games and can separate you from a lot more people that you would rather keep in your life, but when you hate you certainly don't gain. You lose so much respect from others and even more for yourself as you start from becoming bitter to being full of hate.

I think it's maybe that he had a split personality problem where for him to protect himself from being hurt and being the oldest, he felt he had to be the second father in the family and push the rest of us to our limits too. He has to see someone close to him such as me under him, or maybe he's just the kind of person who has to put people down before he can open up to them to realize he can trust them.

Maybe if they hang around for a certain length of time, he will open his barriers to them and show who he can be or is. He could be the one who is more scared of being hurt than anyone as his the one who hurt me. It sometimes makes me wonder if that's why he didn't want to admit to himself that he had a sick brother who needed help but was also capable of looking after himself too. He chose to put me to the side as it would be too hard to go through and making me a target would be much easier same as me putting up my guard to everyone was much easier. That's what I believe he did and accomplished too.

I've also got another younger brother Patrick who I think has a lot in common with me and Patrick is a mystery person who likes to live his separate life in music. He likes to make his own mistakes along the way and not have everyone talk about him too but only as a musician, so he is quite shy to people who say too much. He does have the ability to do anything in music and also has the imagination for it to be realistic and meaningful.

As for my only sister Elizabeth she never gave up on trying to help me and even told me at one stage she was going to study to be a solicitor due to the corrupt chaos people live through here.

Realistically, I just wanted to get as far away as possible from everything and everyone due to my sense of being a problem rather than a person back then. There is also the fact that no one understood however hard they tried because they weren't living it. I didn't want to create any drama at all out of it as I can live with it if people will just leave me alone and stop seeing it as some sort of disease that's going to kill me someday because I could die by just crossing the road and get hit by a car. Just like it is with any other illness.

Because I would have just got on with life if so many people stopped paying so much attention to what I had and just saw who I was instead. I just agreed with whatever Eliza-beth was saying to try and end the conversation even though she was right as I just didn't have any more energy to talk. I always ended up back to square one with how headstrong I was and just knew something I thought were right but not yet been mentioned anywhere in the media as it's all controlled financially, being advised what to do and how to cope with it by others when it was me that was living in an atmosphere. Also, them seeing it on the outside was where the clash was between me and other people who tried to help.

So, from here on, I began hiding everything I felt from them and began to actually hate the thought of talking about anything sensitive and just decided to block anything or conclusive issues coming into my life and just forget battling it and live with anything that comes and let it become a way of life. But I did always have friends, and my family never thought I did as they saw me as a loner due to the quietness I lived at home and the little I showed I knew.

But, I knew a lot more than I let on. All it was, to be honest, was saying nothing at home because I know I'd hear a conversation about it soon by someone else and that it could not be kept at home cause of the worry it might cause. Cause problems are not things to feed off or talk about over and over unless you have first spoken about your problems and solutions to them.

When hard times come, links can be justified from tough problems and no intense thinking will ever be needed as the suffering has already passed and your level of consciousness has already relapsed past this sort of pressure. Now, the wisdom will follow you through to the solutions and solve the problem. After all, nobody wants to live in the past with a life of negativity that always leads to halts or discrimination. On-ly self-pity follows that pathetic lifestyle as the mind is too focused on the one target issue to sustain. Less freedom from the mind is like a corrupt vacation of anxiety, which can break down the nervous system and create the person to have some sort of psychotic breakdown like psychosis if it's not dealt with properly.

Here's an example: some successful men have corrupt thoughts to earn fast, and sustain stability like international bankers who have responsibilities for international systems. In reality, their minds are imprisoned. Some could even be psychopaths or Satanists I think. They never get peace of mind, as greed is never fed. It can never be fed and anxiety follows greed as they've already passed the gluten and materialism lifestyles and are now at the fear of not having everything. Some can even lead to suicide from the rapid change.

I told my close friends everything whenever they were concerned as I'm a person who tells certain people certain things that I know will be safe and sound from strangers who I would never want to tell. Even though strangers are sometimes the best people to talk to, it's the people close to you who are hard to tell as you do not know whether they sometimes are attracted to your difficulties or concerned same as the difference between negative and positive.

I dislike people telling other people my private problems since they don't find it a problem to bring up in a conversation with anyone they know. They don't seem to see any harm in it and it also tells their own life must be incredibly unfulfilled if this is what they end up talking about to still their mind.

When I now look back at all these lessons between me and my older brother, I also see that it was him that may have begun the chapter for me and him to drift apart. Things happen in life to learn respect and earn your needs. Many enemies can be created, but if anything, the lessons would never have a meaning if you never established them like a company doesn't ever get bigger without putting the work into it.

Loneliness can follow any dramatic change in life because not only do you view the world differently, but you also rapidly change inside as your soul moves to another level or your character can move to another purpose maybe. At the end of the day, you gain what you learn from the heart while you memorize and abstract what you learn from the mind. Whatever comes your way or whoever comes your way begin to give a little. Remember to keep your friends and family in life at all times as life's worthless without them and they are always what life is about start to finish. They give a bigger meaning to life than any materialistic or engineered society is capable of trying to achieve.

If a culture can survive to live together with much bigger things than what happened between me and the brother, then countries should be able to survive working with each other and later even continents might be able to work with each other. Finally, the whole world should be able to work together once the systems are all community-based and elite systems are the ones made illegal. The fact they end up becoming psychotic and eventually empires like the EU has become and few ask by who has the EU been funded from the beginning like the Rothschild international bankers. So, try and imagine yourself in a system run by psychopaths, I would rather run my system any day however different I will be seen as because the spirit and the heart are much more powerful than the mind and self-gain like culture is much more powerful than society as it has no label or meaning to it.

Education versus Entrepreneurship

I remember at the age of three I was sent to playschool in Carrighill and can only remember it being in a small cottage across the road from the church where I was baptized. I was the only one sent to playschool after Gerard and Elizabeth for some reason. Shortly after I finished there, the next year I began primary which was only a few minutes walks away from there.

I remember the first day of school all dressed up in my wine uniform, ready to learn whatever was in the system. I did not realize I was actually on a completely different level of learning from what I had ahead of me in my life experiences. This made me start learning from the heart. Thus began the process of me questioning everything twice from a young age if I was not sure it made much sense.

However, the education system I believed had everything to do with the mind and to program people into a system rather than teach them how to behave and be independent later in life. I wondered if this was some sort of mechanism to control us when we should be out as kids having fun and growing up learning about the environment and world we live in more than being stuffed in a room in a uniform.

I never cared about whatever condition I had at this point because I wasn't yet suffering any bit harsh or feeling the effects of it as much as I did when I got older. I had only begun to be skeptical, linking system after system to experience if it didn't make any sense, and wondered what over-rules what. It's just the same as industries that work upon each other and monopolize off each other.

So, in primary in Carrighill, I was quite bored and had no interest in taking part in what we were supposed to be learning, as I felt these kinds of things we probably already know in our subconscious, such as the 'ABC' or numbers.

Same as in today's world, a child can go work on the Internet where before you'd have to have some sort of qualification to be able to work online and so on.

So, for anything I felt was not useful, I linked the ignorance of people allowing it to be continued while working by ego. I knew nothing about the way the education system was controlled and that this might also be the problem with the system been broken.

Here's something I did question a lot. I saw my parents struggle hard during the eighties recession and when they were trying to paint a picture that school is a great thing, I was wondering why they were still struggling if they had already been there.

They were the kind of things I had in mind even though I was only a child. No matter how the side effects were affecting me as I developed, I was also achieving the same level of the bigger picture to view to wake up to the real world and what it's like out there, rather than continue to be trained to be ready for it later. So everything was going fine in the first few years. I was learning all the basics and how to communicate with others until I began to act up on things due to the emotional bullying by Gerard at home and when I had no contact with Ciara anymore after he had told me where to tell her to go. I became more lost in myself. Things changed in me rapidly after this and I became more unforgiving towards anything that happened and more lost in the system of school as emotion had now passed out my consciousness.

I lost interest in wanting to go home after school too because I didn't want to be near Gerard for I wanted to avoid having any tension with him. I also became insecure about where I stood in the class and wondered, "Was I soon going to be treated here like I am at home by Gerard and his tactics?"

I really wanted to be a good person but was being pushed further and further every time I tried to fit in at home, so I soon began to turn on everyone who even tried to get close to me. I became very aggressive if someone tried to manipulate me or trick me or even tell me what to do as my consciousness was already beginning to be manipulated with medications, which was never believed possible at this stage as they were believed only to get people better.

I had already been told what to do in school, but I was behaving in school according to the way things were going on at home or anywhere else, making me act up without me subconsciously realizing it. In that sense, I became the bully in school from being misunderstood at home and pushed around and felt frowned upon because of what I had. My goal was now to block everyone from my life and not let anyone get the better of me, even when they were not trying to, and especially block those that were trying to help me. I caused problem after problem for myself very quickly by taking on the whole class who I thought was going to turn on me as Gerard did at home. I would be more ready for what I have to face if that was the case in the long run and build up this big wall that was a complete waste of time. It was the eighties so industries and companies were facing rapid decreases in all directions, and poverty and ignorance were the same way as society or economies decline.

It was time to toughen up. Epilepsy and life were beginning to become more of a journey to survive than get through, so I was in some way able to link to how the recession had hit people's lives from the beginning to emotionally suffering a condition being mass medicated for, which is how the heart works by its silent brain and directs information to the brain.

The country in my consciousness was becoming preoccupied with a different atmosphere! The people in primary were not much of a problem at all. Most problems were self-inflicted because at this age that's how we learn; by making mistakes, but I could not forgive what Gerard had done to me because I was not as fulfilled as I used to be with Ciara anymore and now she was completely gone for good.

I got into situations to guard myself against more people. I can't remember anyone who gave me a bad time in primary school through those years. Everyone was there for one another. But, I did give some people there a hard time when I was walked over or targeted or even played with, which I do regret today because I took out any rage I had at home on Gerard in school to whoever got in my way.

I became a kid who had built up serious issues and wanted to be in control of everything. The fact that the one person who used to fulfill me was gone, I was labeled with something I couldn't control, along with dangerous medications I couldn't describe the effects of. My consciousness became over-active with thoughts of being left out of the family system because I not telling them what was wrong with me. I didn't tell them because I was already telling them the truth about what the drugs had been doing to my consciousness, and they felt I was looking for attention or self-pity. So after telling about the effects so many times and running out of ways to tell them any other way, I stopped telling them altogether. I spent as much time as possible away from home, but can also understand now that my parents had five kids to look after and couldn't always get everything right. I used to read the effects of each medication I took as I got older and saw numerous effects they could cause when I was only taking them to stop myself from having seizures.

This thought pattern became very big in my consciousness. Much of what I learned growing up made no sense to me and I felt more like been programmed. I kept thinking maybe I have to make myself more noticed like someone who was looking for directions to get somewhere. Out of stupidity and keeping everything in, I wanted Gerard to know nothing about me anymore after what he had done.

I told no family member anything even if I was forced to because I knew he would find another way of getting the better of me. I did a real good job of keeping things from family members but in a bad way, which destroyed me from learning properly due to the pressure I put on myself. What I should have been focusing on, when I look back now, was that I see a different me that had put up loads of walls at a very young age and saw way too soon how the real world can be.

A few years after that, in fourth class, I was out of control with my behavior, scared of absolutely nothing. But inside, I was a good and loyal person, promising myself not to fail in life, but wasn't opening up to anyone. But I did have one particular friend, John Sheen, who was about three miles away. I cycled to his place regularly, and he would come to mine too, and I could tell him what was wrong as he would not tell anyone else. He was the same age as me and Nigel, who I began to know through my parents being friends with his parents. I came to visit at weekends but was living too far away to become friendlier with him.

However, when I was eleven, we moved five miles away and bought a pub, and changed schools. I was gutted and didn't want to move anywhere as I believed I've built my spot here now. No one was giving me a hard time at school even though it was nearly the end of primary. I was very worried about how I was going to fit into another school but also knew that maybe it won`t be as bad, as I learned that not all people are like Gerard. We weren't moving that far from some friends I had and it was closer to Nigel too, so I was okay with it after a while and was looking forward to living above a public house.

I started going to a school a few minutes' walks up the road from the pub where we had moved. Life began to become a lot busier with living over a pub and having my mum manage it. My dad was still working for himself at the same time and would come back from work and do more work in the pub to give my mum a break and so on.

I was seeing all the time and effort the price of living was doing to them and it was a hectic life for them. I was still questioning why they were living like this when they are both educated and went to college and so on. In this new school, there was a bully called Shane, just like any other school has one or two, and he began to show me on the first day I went that he was the boss in and I was to be aware of it, by being sarcastic and smart to my face. I just looked at him and laughed because I was not scared of anyone, or nobody for that matter, after the challenges I had got in my life thus far. So whoever wanted a go-off with me, no matter how big they were, would get a challenge back. I wouldn't back down because I was already bruised inside from putting up with the tricks and manipulations while growing up, wondering if I would ever get better. So, if someone wanted to have a go at me, they were welcome to try it; if not, this was even better at that stage.

I and Shane were more or less getting into fights almost every day for one whole year in school and even after school. We couldn't stand the sight of each other; I'd lash out at him anytime I saw him, and he would lash out on me anytime he saw me. When I look back now, it was a part of growing up. We suddenly came to a stop and just called it quits on both sides before one of us ended up more hurt than the other. We began to talk more than fight and still got into the odd fight now and then, but not as much, and became good mates in the end.

We usually look back at primary and more or less laugh at it or salute each other if we ever see each other later in life as we came to understand knowing where we stood with each other. We had met our match for all the years we were at others, with me in Carrighill and him in Saleen, which was the name of the place we moved to.

Soon, we had moved on to secondary school in Dun Lock in Cork, where I wasn't in a hurry to forget about at all. Shortly after finishing primary, I chose to go to secondary there, which was also a college because girls went there too. I presumed I might get in there sometime, so I went in with my mother to see the school and saw a place in the gym in there that had a climbing wall above it with loads of other facilities.

I ran up and wanted to have a go at it and wasn't allowed because there were too many people around, so I just walked around to see how high it was and wanted to climb to the very top of it. I went to see it when there was room and loved it. Then, as I turned around to walk out of there, I bumped into Nigel who was also thinking of picking this school and for the same reasons too, so we caught up with each other and decided we would both pick this school by the looks of it. We both surprisingly ended up in the same class after the exam we attempted to see what level would suit us. I had very little understanding at this time of where it was leading me to go though. Even though I wanted to do well in everything, I just couldn't think straight that I needed to go to these places and learn with interest rather than thinking of getting out of the place as soon as possible or even studying anything without daydreaming.

I just had no interest in the system that I knew was going to be of least value to me later in life when reality had already been in my life about how the real world can be. All I was interested in doing was getting successful so that I could be of some help to my parents and hopefully won't have to go through the same pressure of living as they were.

I was constantly thinking about trying to come up with new ideas. Nothing was coming to mind just yet even though I was also tortured by the drugs all along, so I tried to fit into the class at one stage. They were a messy crowd who had no value of the interest in anything they were learning besides messing and having fun. So, I said to myself, This is not going to be any bit helpful at all. The messing continued.

I started to get my first seizure in there and right away I was targeted with a nickname (Electric Eddie) which was ok at the start, but I got mocked with it every day soon as it was my nickname in school and many would be reminding me of when the next seizure will start.

One day a guy who had shown his true colors in there shouted out Electric Eddie and I didn't answer or look at him. He did it again, so I told him to shut up. Then he did it again. I got up, threw his table down on the floor, and said quit the name-calling. Then, that was the worst thing I had ever done like half of the class copied him after seen that, took on his role, and started calling me the same name. I knew I let myself in for a very serious problem with the class then.

Things then started to get very tensed in secondary very quickly. I began to hate it more than anything and became sicker having to go in there five days a week as I was getting more depressed with trying to be good at things like art, metal work, and woodwork that I enjoyed but couldn't learn properly with not been able to ignore the name-calling and continuing to get seizures in a class like that.

This began to make me more tired or dosed-up and that increased getting mocked even more by some of the class. I started to become more violent every time, lashing out at everyone mocking me because I used to stand my ground no matter how big the person was. For something I have that I can't control and plays a large role in how I fit in with society and being mocked and harassed about it was not exactly linked to being able to learn greatly in school. I never walked away from people who enjoyed having a go at other people like me back then because they're the people who need a very serious wake-up call, so there was a battle for first place going on at this stage.

Each time I got mocked, I fought back no matter how big the crowd was as they were a gang of their own. Sometimes I succeeded, and sometimes I got beaten up, which to be honest I'm glad in some ways I did because I was getting payback for the way I had behaved in primary and what comes around always goes around. My time was simply up. It was now time for me to learn the hard way in many ways, so I did as I had to.

So, after the second year in the dun lock, people were already leaving this class being expelled due to drinking alcohol numerous times or smoking in class, fighting in class, and even throwing tools around that we weren't allowed to use in the end due to the behavior, so there was no learning system here at all. I wanted to move to another class but was told I'd have to go back a year to be allowed to do that and that was fine with me. I said, "I would." I just wanted out from the previous class to see if I could learn anything I would fit into.

The next year, I began the second year again as I had learned absolutely nothing in the last class. The new class was up a few levels from the last one and more intelligent and a lot more easy-going, things improved very well for a while as in months and I began to feel more confident on fitting in somewhere until a girl who had no interest in anything started to annoy me looking for my attention.

I didn't get it as I learned from giving attention the first time I ended up twice as bad and she began to tell tales to the teachers that I was annoying her, pushing her and all those small things which were lies at the time as I just ignored her and other stupid little things like I was saying something about her that's not true, and sure that eventually had me kick off a fuss. I told her where to go and said, "Go away home to wherever you belong if you're going to be like this!:

She caused up another stir when I said that and began to tell people that I said bad things about her place, which was pathetic because it's Carrighill where I went to primary, so it made no sense. I was annoyed and went to the teacher Mr. Fitzgerald a few hours later who had told me when I started going to school here to come to him whenever I had a problem as he was also the social worker.

As I did have a problem here, two and a half years on after, he helped me move out of the previous class I did not like. I told him that a girl in my new class is telling people from her town Carrighill where I first went to primary a lot of lies about me saying things about it when I went to primary there, where she's more or less trying to get my attention and I'm going to go crazy if she won't just leave me alone. He was in the middle of doing something; going through files while listening to me and said he doesn't want to know and can't I see he's very busy right now so don't worry about it is what he said and I'm sure things will be ok.

I looked at him and said you're the one that asked me to come if anything was bothering me! He said he was too busy right now and told me to go back to class because the break is almost over. Then I started to get angry and lost my temper cause I was doing what he asked me to do and being shown the door, so I acted up and caught a chair and threw it a few feet away to the other side of the room. I was getting fired up with rage and wanted to take my anger out on him after he told me to come to talk to him if something's wrong which is exactly what I had done but he was not interested as he had too much going on which I couldn't fully accept at fifteen.

Then shut the door and told me to stay put while I was angry. Then I just wanted to go home, so I walked to the door. He stopped me from going out and told me to sit down or he will sit me down himself. I didn't so he caught me and pinned me up to the wall, giving me a wake-up call, so I told him to let me go. I pushed him away as hard as I could and just sat down and knew that was the end of secondary school for me and began to feel left out again. I had just accepted that I was not supposed to be in a system at this time that most others are.

He rang my mother to collect me, and I asked him, "Is that it now for me in secondary? Am I getting expelled for losing my temper due to the fact I did what I was asked and needed the guidance of where I was being led when you didn't fully have the time for it?" And he simply replied, "Yes, Eddie, maybe so. But you've got away with enough now at this stage."

He brought me into the vice principal's office and told her what happened that I had acted up again☐was not doing what I was told. She turned to my mum when my mum arrived and said, "Your son needs psychological help and we don't have it here for people with his behavior and again nobody was any bit awake to the main thing that was bordering me all along here which was the side effects from medications."

That made me feel very low right where I started again and that I had disappointed my mother, I felt alone, confused, and isolated from everyone again. I had not belonged here in this environment either. That was my last day at Dun Lock Secondary School; I was only fifteen.

Mr. Fitzgerald has today gone into politics after he left his job as a teacher a few years later. After leaving school, I became self-destructive on myself more than ever for letting my parents down with what I had first and now this too. And the education system in Ireland's culture was incredibly important to back then which it still is and leaving was never an option whatever problems you had or whether it worked out for you or not.

There wasn't anything I could do if I wasn't going to learn from the lack of work that was done from people's messing and other forms of manipulation. I was not the only person who felt failed by the system either for personal reasons. My personal and common seizures were just too much at this time to fit into this learning program for society, while I was also developing and on four different types of medications taking up to fifteen pills a day that I felt could not be healthy at all.

After leaving school, I came to terms I am on my own whether I like it or not. I immediately began looking for work at local companies and building sites, but I was too young and knew I'd find it difficult with epilepsy. My parents were completely disgusted with me getting kicked out, but they were not there to see how it had failed me, what had happened and that I was not the only person this happened to either. They expected me to be like any other normal child with the challenges and experiences that were a part of my life path in the first place, I would have tried a lot harder if I felt I was being treated more normal or listened to, but I had more downfalls to deal with that I never agreed to experience. That had pressured me to go my way to survive from the very beginning without me planning it to be that way.

A lot had built up to common sense why I was acting up so differently. Even though they are my parents and always meant well and thought they knew much more than me because I was only a kid and have not grown up yet, does not mean the current systems they grew up with have not changed or will be as relevant when our generation grows up. However, I did learn what the real world and people are like very quickly that changed my strategies of how I wanted to live my life too in some ways.

The biggest problem at home was Gerard and every time I tried to explain to my parents that he was annoying me, "Which would remind me of what he had done with Ciara when I was young", he would try and turn the story around that there are two sides to every story. The fact that I was hard work due to my outbursts is also very true but I was hard work for a reason like I was in school too. Also, the fact I already had something I could not control in my life I was not going to be mistreated in other places.

Gerard turned around to my mum soon after I left school and said, "What's he going to do now?" My mum began a conversation with him as if I had killed somebody, was on my way to prison and it made me feel sick to the stomach hearing her explain everything to Gerard where realistically he only wanted to hear all that so he could wind me up more.

I soon began looking for a major structure in my life to plan my way of leaving home and decided to begin washing cars for people while they were having a drink in the public house, shortly after a building that I wanted to put up a sign for it to expand. But, my mum wouldn't allow me since it was not a real business or insured, so then I thought logically after about a year of doing this and wondered if there was any chance of getting a loan to buy a drive-through car wash that I could pay off monthly and earn something from. Where it may also bring more business to the public house, especially for short-time drinkers, who will come for that particular reason and earn me something and the parents more customers.

Getting that type of machine at this time was just a dream so I got a small second-hand power washer and used that for a while. It kept me busy and made me feel more secure than I felt in school at something. I knew I needed more opportunities to open up. This is only short-term to getting my place and making money, so I went back to the drawing board and wondered what else I could do and soon began to valet cars too along with washing them, so I was beginning to think big and take full control of my goal.

My parents could see the after-effects that I was a lot happier with myself and better off out of the school system at this point and I was a lot happier to see them calmer than before with less worrying involved.

About two years after leaving school, I met the girl from the class who was annoying me that time I changed class. I met her out in a local nightclub with her partner and she came over to me, wanting to apologize after what happened in school. She said that she was only messing with me then and did not expect things to get so carried away at the time. I didn't care as much then as I did before and accepted the apology since I didn't feel school worked out for me then either with what was already going on in my life.

I'm also a middle child and sometimes wondered whether it was middle-child syndrome characteristics I may have had as I never fully felt a part of the family or where I stood probably because of shutting Gerard out very early in life after what he had done and never forgiving him. I always felt like the problem from then rather than finding the solution to the problem.

Even though I had loving parents who wanted the best for all of us, I could be my own worst enemy too being as stubborn as I was and not wanting any help from anyone anymore unless they understood me since that did not work the last time I had asked for it, which made things more difficult for the parents with me wanting to do it all alone since I felt alone. I wanted to be everything I could and prove everyone who had to doubt me wrong and succeed in everything I knew at only that age since I felt let down in other ways already. But as stubborn as I was, I wouldn't tell them that because I didn't want to advertise myself to everyone like the time I heard my mum talk to Gerard.

So, I felt if I opened my mouth about something, everyone might soon know and I don't mean that in a bad way. I think it's the fact I felt alone for so long at this point too that my views and needs changed. I would not have been able to handle that level of attention all of a sudden because I didn't want it anymore after what had happened with Gerard to what had happened in dun lock school. I had turned against need in life and put it more towards work. So, listening to or hearing people talk about me became more annoying than helpful. I began to put more time into work and decided that I would start going around to people's houses doing what I was doing in the car park of the public house.

I also moved on and began to do window cleaning too. This had simply started with me walking with a bucket five to six miles every Saturday with a few tools in it calling to people's homes and having no bike or transport since I was not allowed to drive due to the seizures anyway. I had saved up and managed to get a bike the following Christmas which made that routine every weekend a lot more simple than it was and I had finally got my name around Cork in those few years of doing that and managed to begin to travel around Cork and Ireland too, As I got older□eighteen □everything got more difficult. This was due to the fact I couldn't drive as we were entering a new technical world where everything became more mobile and societies along with the world began to communicate quicker than ever.

I wasn't any good with technology and couldn't understand how it worked. Everyone began to get mobile phones and create businesses much faster than before. My biggest loss was I couldn't be mobile because I couldn't drive, so I planned to open a garage in the back of the car park in the pub and see if I could buy a car wash drive-through again and go from there. Suddenly, all that came to a stop because after having the public house a few years we were moving house away from Saleen just a mile down the road and selling the pub and the new owner wasn't too keen to let me continue what I was doing fulltime, which is understandable.

So, I had to call an end to that from there which I had learned by now that everything must come to an end, but I continued to go away with the bucket on the bike every Saturday to customers a few more miles away at this stage. I began to feel that I wasn't getting anywhere doe after nearly another year of this and having full-time jobs I had started the following two years where one was landscaping and gardening and the other was working in a precast making all types of concrete products. Doing these jobs and while continuing doing my jobs, I had decided to put a stop to washing cars and windows.

The seizures were coming upon me more frequently than before too☐I began to get more tired and a little depressed. From there on, after another six months, I was bored again and didn't want to be in a precast yard any longer so I began searching for work I previously enjoyed, which I got quite quickly. I first got a job in Brosnons garage near Cork city washing cars again, and this lasted about six months.

The main problem again here was the fact I had no transport and it took me an hour to get there and go home every day due to that. I used to hitch up and down every day or get the bus as far as I could and walk the rest of the way. The fact it was a bit out from the main road, I had to be aware of this while coming back from there every night.

I used to pass another place a few miles down which was on the main road and closer to the city, which transports cars around the country, and said to myself, If I could get in there it would be better because I could see more structure there and more long-term demand, so that was my next step. I looked them up on the yellow pages called powers transport, rang them up explaining that I have been washing cars for years myself and who I was with. After I stopped□but didn't tell him anything about the seizures I was getting□he asked how many I could do in a day. I said around thirty and he said to come up for a few weeks trial next week; it started from there.

It wasn't washing them in powers I was doing doe. It was de-waxing all the vehicles because they came straight in from the ships that were importing them from abroad and were full of wax to stop them from rusting from the seawater on the journey over. The conversation went down fine and for the next few months, I fitted in with the rest of the team there who were my age and older from the city. My main problem again was having no transport and no one knowing why, but I didn't tell them why I couldn't drive because I knew I would be discriminated against in no time.

However, I knew something had to give way and I got tired of it after six months and left because my dad had said I can work with him if I want, which is in construction, and had told me this a few times already. I wasn't sure about it first because working with family can be very different from working with work-mates, same as blood is thicker than water. But I also felt at the same time I had nothing to lose and everything to gain. I didn't have to hide the fact I was getting seizures either or didn't have a transport problem, so I said "Okay, sure, why not."

Everything was fine at the start. He gave me space after telling me what he wanted to be done and left me alone. As time went by, but I could see much easier ways and quicker ways of him finishing jobs and starting others sometimes expect that was not my responsibility and he had been at it a lot longer and knew the routine of doing it his ways.

I always gave myself a deadline when I began something. And months later, things got quiet, and all I was doing was going out to the van and getting stuff for him and my interest in this work began to get a little quieter than it had been. This brought on fear and anxiety to me of how much pressure he was under to look after his family and how does he survive when things get a little quiet like they were at this time. I began to try and think of ways to try and expand. As father and son, we got on pretty good for working and living together even though I also became more depressed than ever.

I felt I was getting older and had to earn more and was more worried about been better too. But, I didn't want to let him down either. I did lose interest in the occupation, a level of which was caused by depression which says☐de-pressure☐when you divide it.

I think he more or less knew that anyway because one time when I was at my lowest in Cork Mental Centre, changing anti-depressants, another brother of mine was looking for work and my father said he will take him on for now until I get better and see how things go with him.

I was fine with that as I also wanted something new and creative to find too so it worked out well for both of us and from there on, I was at home often thinking and thinking. Then, all of a sudden, one day I thought of the day I began to draw, which was when my dog I got for my sixth birthday had died from been knocked down and I was deeply sad because I only had him a few days.

I remembered that day I started to draw and always knew I had the talent but more or less had to be in the mood for it and never put any more effort into it. So, I started all that creative interest up again since I had to focus on becoming better anyway and used this as therapy too. The more I did it, the more I surprised myself. It helped me heal a lot of bitter feelings and negative behavior I had blocked. I had something to look at that I did, which was even better. I knew these talents were in me but just didn't give myself the time to create anything. The ability was always there. My parents were always telling me to go further with it, but I lacked interest due to working all the time-traveling and becoming depressed later throughout the years, and felt I could easily get bored later. This time, once I started I kept at it, but I also wanted to make money out of it or make some sort of image to what I'm creating if that makes any sense. I began to take my drawings to tattoo artists as that was my next plan to get into tattooing and art was the only occupation I knew I would stick to for a long period and was more or less the only thing I had one hundred percent patience for and enjoyed at the same time.

But, that idea of tattooing only filled the gap for a while, so I began to paint shortly after that with all different types of paints. I got the hang of it very quickly and it also began helping me out of this deep depression I was locked in. I used to paint ideas I had in my head straight onto the canvas, which for me at the time made everything complete and cleared the negativity around me. Everything surrounding me became alive. It was nice to see something complete that my consciousness had thought of and that created me to feel fulfilled. I began doing paintings more or less every day, and I believe the more I did, the more it deteriorated the depression and I began to finally gain more confidence for once in a very long time.

I knew I had artistic talents and design talents. I wanted to aim a lot higher like I did before and began to ask myself what exactly can I give that I have and I said self-help! As with all my previous knowledge on how the world and problems are created,

So the first thing I wanted to do, is finding out how countries work with one another, and the fact that America and the United Kingdom have always been powerhouses, I began researching about failures like health systems and mental institutes and prisons and countries depts. Since I had fully been involved in some of them. I also went back to the Routh on the time Independence Day began in some countries and asked myself, how did they begin to create an industrial materialistic country so fast with fewer people living there then than now and manage to merge with the other powerful countries again so soon? Where did the structure begin so quickly? Are the banks created with loans that don't exist to create debts for people to get into debt and work their life`s away for the people who engineered this structure in the first place at a basic income? Education is meant to be a tool for guidance and creativity in the real world where today it is more about keeping you away from the real world and suppressing you into a false world of peace and success with point-scoring in materialism been the maintenance system for the elites.

Along with some qualifications that mean nothing. Ask yourself this. Europe's greatest monuments, oldest buildings, bridges, caves, tunnels; Egypt's pyramids — who built them? People with college qualifications? People in debt? Or people who had their sovereignty thinking for themselves? And today over one trillion of America's debt is from college fees with not all of the people holding on to this debt promised very good career paths at all.

Many people don't realize we're built to create anything we want if we want it. It's like if you were out on an island stuck alone like the film "Cast Away" would you find a way to build a boat? Damn, right you would. As creation never leaves the consciousness as the sub consciousness is always communicating to it and humans are made to adapt to any level of operating to survive.

Depression

Depression can be a silent killer in a twenty-four hour seven day a week tree hundred and sixty-five day a year raw atmosphere, that deteriorates your body and consciousness. It's like two worlds have collided a way of life into a living self-destructive consciousness. More importantly, only you can educate your way out of it step by step. You can either learn from it or drown yourself down a path so far that the beginning of suicidal thoughts will follow one way or another. If it's grounded at a deep level for a long period it makes the person unaware of a way out. I think it has a sort of negative storm effect on someone, and the problem in today's world is people who write books on depression don't all write them for people in depression but for people who want to know about it.

For example, a depressed individual whose consciousness is shattered and self-esteem is exhausted picks up a book written about depression and they question everything in the book that doesn't fit into their situation at all because there are so many different types of it and all there looking for is a way out of it. It can be more of an emotional journey than an illness.

It's very difficult for someone depressed to understand when they're self-destructive like it is for a racing driver to realize what speed they could be

126

doing. You have to win their understanding to help them, same as people who fall in love win each other's hearts and trust. People with depression doubt themselves way too much due to their low level of self-esteem to feeling emotionally stressed from exhaustion to thinking negative that's manipulating their consciousness. In the long term, madness follows where insanity can sometimes occur when their mental health starts to deteriorate along with psychosis.

But, I also believe from experience that depression is not an illness at all, but a suppressed condition. If you look at the word, it says depression□which also says the pressure□and if you've lived through the condition and overcame it, you'll realize it's also a constant emotion that dictates how you behave and feel.

The longer you stay in it, I believe the longer you'll be able to connect to lower dimensions and emotions and realize how your heart also has its brain, which is raw and incredibly torturing emotions. Some say these are also the dimensions you go to if you do bad things like commit suicide or are a bad person in general who was aware of the bad things they did in life and so on but continued to live that path anyway.

So here's another thing; imagine the people who are in power. I mean real people in power who are elites such as some international bankers and bondholders and shareholders etc. Just imagine what pressure they have every day trying to keep that position in the developed world for their benefit.

There's a saying that "Power corrupts, but absolute power corrupts." So imagine you being one of these people for a very long time like throughout a career of forty years, and you'll be probably closer to someone who can be called a complete psychopath or whose mental health must be shattered from being behind the game in power. If you were not using this power for the right reasons because you got your way for years and still are not fulfilled like greed never has enough, you become more fulfilled seeing others worse off than you or at least joining whatever system you create.

If you think about it, someone like this would have absolutely no interest in making the world a better place, but as I said about the dimensions earlier, those types of people would also only be linked to make the world reach those horrible dimensions.

They would be out of power if the world was the opposite in peace and harmony which most people in the world need anyway. Also, their out of power anyway with them trying to enslave humanity in financial debt that's only created out of fresh air from many private banks in the first place with their minds slaved to the systems creating it.

Your goal should be to find gradually your way out of this system and into another view of life that will be more fulfilling "It's all down to whom you are and why you're in this zone of distress to how your depressed condition was caused." People need to realize that being fed up with things is so much more different from depression and they can never relate comparing themselves to those in that situation unless they have been there before.

When you're fed up, your logical way of thinking can restructure your methods and still be able to satisfy whatever needs you to have. When you're depressed, it doesn't matter how you want something because all you want is a way out of this drained atmosphere zone that's pulled you away from society and driven you to a disturbed mind of tormenting thoughts to harbor your consciousness and make you feel you deserve all this pain and you're nothing and become isolated.

If anything, you shouldn't be even breathing so you're self-destructive and you feel it all the time where you should be the opposite. You should be free, loving, and love yourself first. But, when you are depressed love is the illusion when you're in love depression can be the illusion.

It's basically like a lower self-eating you up piece by piece and your consciousness drifts away from the current reality to isolation from the rest of society. It can't adapt to any current neutral way of life anymore and everything becomes a lot slower and more awkward. You begin to neglect yourself, your family, and your friends as you lose your way of thinking and can't explain how you feel anymore. Nothing seems to look positive anymore whatever you are told.

Then, at the same time, all you begin to see are big things in front of you as if you were shrinking or are like a child seeing houses. The world has got much bigger because you have suppressed your way of thinking. All of a sudden, you drift into nothing and believe you're nothing and feel you have died because your spirit has where what's just happened there, in the long run, is that you went from being in society to out of society due to depression.

There are people on the streets in this state every single day, but due to the speed we've grown up and the speed of living in society, these people tend to be ignored or classed as nobodies in the world were in since the twenty-first-century in the developed world.

If everyone inflated could just place themselves in their shoes for just one day, maybe they would learn that there is not much difference between the man on the streets and the flashy businessman or businesswoman with a massive corporation built.

The fact is that these people just don't have the same identity at the same time even though both link off each other. These are people who are fighting an inflated system of guilt or destruction due to their way of thinking and their way of living and if you were one of them, why would you want to come back to society when you then see how much distance the ignorance we allow drifts from a world of materials to a world of reality.

I was in that world from age eighteen to twenty-two on and off, and my consciousness was so far gone at nineteen and became worse in the end that someone could convince me that black was white and white was black or pigs could fly and the strength between believing something and knowing by intuition was also gone.

You believe you're nothing when you're this low, and you don't even know you're depressed either. In some cases, that's how so many suicides don't seem to register with their friends or family. It's a fact of self-punishment due to all this consciousness madness where the person just snaps, not realizing what they're even going through or about to do.

Our health system used to be out of structure here in Ireland with a population of over 4.5 million and the treatment the disabled get was and still is someway disgraceful due to our lack of patience and knowledge of some of these conditions. Disability is a reality along being materialistic is an illusion. A perfect example is: let's say you were depressed like I'm explaining. How are you meant to go to a doctor and understand the questions there asking you like how you're feeling? What are you thinking of doing? If anything, the only way to provide evidence is to write down a day's thinking for a week on how you feel and what you're thinking of doing including interests, which is another thing that's very slack while depressed due to the so-called chemical imbalance which has no scientific facts.

Our moods reflect on the way we think and then bring an effect on us. That's solid evidence because like I said earlier, while depressed it's very difficult to fit in anywhere with society no matter where you go or who you are. That includes understanding and fitting in because writing includes your thoughts of failure that you feel and thoughts of isolation and it can make the psychologist judge your department of depression and go from there. I felt so out of touch and alone and isolation and depression led me to rock bottom that the emptiness made me feel more like an object out of this world. This was not anything new and thoughts of suicide soon appeared after feeling this way for so long.

I honestly believe I would be long gone today only for my family and friends and especially my mother because whatever way I thought, she always got me on the right path whether she understood me or not. It just didn't matter. She was always there to help, and I felt pathetic that I couldn't help myself out of this mess on my own at times. The stubbornness took a toll and made me beat myself up even more that I needed help or someone on my side. It was as if I had these voices in my head telling me that I'm scum and should seriously think of ending my life as soon as possible if I know what's better for me.

This was realistically the deterioration of one way of consciousness snapping from normality to mental. Soon after that, my mental health did go. I had a total breakdown and had not cried for over three years, as I didn't feel I could due to the damage the mind and medications had caused. I was all shattered and battered from no fear of anything.

After the poor quality of life and after so much neglect, anyone goes into isolation and doesn't feel anything but sour and poor neglect. Twisted feelings begin to erupt from frustration and don't want any part of the world you've been brought up in as it feels like the whole world has got so big and you're so lost and can't see any bit of structure coming into your life anymore. You see everyone else get on with their lives creates guilt from your failure, and you just don't know where to turn, so all of the sudden neglect turns to give up, and boredom shortly follows after that.

You dwell on things that you shouldn't have done or what if and maybe this that, but realistically why not say to yourself that if we were all the same logical thinkers and had the same structure of life, we would live in a pretty boring society. If anything, being different or separate should feel more challenging with more options to create success and be unique.

Thinking negatively about everything, forgetting about any good things that happened, and not finding any way of communicating with any bit of normality in your life can come to a halt for so long that you'll create a structural demand for failure as you make yourself believe you're a failure. So, if anyone thinks like this, then get out of there before it's too late. Otherwise, when depression follows, it will be a terrifying battleground. It will take longer to return to your true self.

I turned into someone who was scared of nothing when I came to this stage because I wanted out. I had just this small bit of demand towards myself from the failure of being any bit successful due to the things I was not allowed to do but had done anyway. This is what kept me alive along with getting this far in life.

I walked down the most dangerous parts of Cork at three a.m. and four a.m. at nineteen years of age and nobody ever bothered me when I was hoping to be finished off or just beaten up at times to feel anything. The same happened in Dublin and Limerick whenever I went on my travels and even London! Maybe people could sense I was not scared of anything or there was something wrong with me taking all these risks when others would never dare.

The only reason was that my life was a mess anyway, so I had nothing to lose and if people did try and wrestle me to the ground at that time, they were only going to be doing me a favor. All I wanted to feel was something again and the reason I wanted that was to feel normal for once because with depression and medication effects like I said earlier, you begin to feel like an object. No sensation alerts in your body anymore, which is why people lose their sex drive during it. The only thing that ever works is instinct. At the same time, I didn't look for it but felt safe where it was because it opened my consciousness back to reality.

However stupid it may sound, I felt a lot safer in dangerous places than I did at home because when you're at this stage, still trying to fit into what's normal, your sense of feeling any bit normal is gone. The danger becomes a need to make you realize you still are in control, so when your senses work, it makes you feel some way normal.

Whether you're rich or someone with a great job, someone who has a happy lifestyle, someone whose done everything by the book, it doesn't matter what you are; depression can affect anyone at any time of their lives whatever society they grew up in or are growing up in. Never take anything for granted because too many already do.

It has to do with how you think and where you are in life, and it's silent but the fact is you can't be helped with it until you admit you have it where a lot of people don't even know they have it. They accept the fact that you will need to be helped in some way to get out of it, and hopefully when you do, you will never get it again, which most don't if they can find a lifestyle to keep them away from it. People want to be active and begin to trust people to create a different atmosphere in their life rather than isolating themselves from everything and everyone because they feel left out and again as it is a complete mind game.

The mind is an unnatural time bomb that we have to try and communicate with it to neutralize our belief and thought structure and create positive situations in society. There is nothing more powerful than the mind like there is nothing bigger than the universe. It creates everything you lose and everything you gain.

The only way to explain how silent and dangerous it is is by comparing the power of mother nature on planet Earth to the power of consciousness. Storms and earthquakes can just come along and wipe out cities that then must be rebuilt again. When you're in a bad state of consciousness, it will play serious games with you like when I was in depression for so long. It created negativity and the consciousness became overactive that I couldn't control everything around me or couldn't understand how anything worked anymore.

I was like a child learning all over again. Everything looked so big, and I felt as slow as a snail and sometimes nearly had panic and anxiety attacks trying to fit in again, and that's how isolation kept me drifting away from others. I was a complete mess and I remember sometimes going up to Cork for the day. Which was not that far away, but it felt so far away due to the depression because I didn't like being at home too long when I wasn't understood. I already moved out before and didn't want to isolate myself more there, but no one is to blame for that. I didn't have any communication skills for anyone at home to understand me or my situation, but I had to try some way to stay motivated. I was also out of work for a year at this time during the times I was going up to Dublin every few months for tests.

Time had taken its toll, and I just couldn't see any way forward from all the medications and continued side effects and seizures. I felt useless being out of work. I felt isolated having no one understand me and I felt lonely being alone in this monopolized game with so much frustration building up in me and very little love even though I'd a lot to give and a lot who loved me.

I had way too many issues in the situation I was caught up in and didn't even look for a woman because I used to say to myself I was too pathetic to be with one and don't deserve one and again this was my dark consciousness with a voice in my head telling me I'm no good and don't deserve to be happy and this torture will never end because I deserve to be punished.

Sometimes I would hit myself in the head wishing I could control my consciousness from these overwhelming experiences. I was in a horrible state not see any way out of any path I managed to plot into it was like a dominos effect of darkness. I was just in a state of dark roads where nothing looked possible and I used to test myself as I felt no way normal or could not feel anything anymore. One day in Cork, I saw a car coming and deliberately stepped out before it came and crossed the road, but I felt I had to do it to remind me that I can in some way still feel the normality of living. It was not right beside me but made me feel I had to get to the other side of the road fast, so it was more or less to test my sense. It made me feel a small bit normal again for a short period.

I used to analyze everyone who looked so happy and wondered how they were and what made them this happy. Then I wished I could be like them, but my consciousness just didn't adjust to show me that way. I used to just look into the river so often wanting to throw myself in there mostly again from side effects, but the water is something that heals me so quick and stops the negative thinking for just a few minutes, so I used to spend a lot of time near the sea and test my consciousness. I wanted to see whether it was time to go or stick around for another.

I was out in a boat before and managed to get a seizure and almost drowned only for my friend Liam catching me in the water and pulling me back up by the lace of my boot. At the time, he was not able to swim so how was it my time to go when he had just saved my life along with everything else I was experiencing? How you think your life is structured and how people get into being depressed is not something that happens overnight. Some might have it for years and not even realize it while others decide to stay in denial about it. This is because they don't believe the case that normal people can get it too and would rather they stay in denial than get help for it, as they don't feel they would have a life anymore by getting help.

There's a true saying: 'the worst has got to happen before the best even though the help for it can also be a complete waste of time too sometimes.' But, that's fair enough too if they're too stubborn or scared to change because many people don't like facing up to reality and stay in a false comfort zone where they feel they belong. I, for one, would try and do try everything possible to get rid of it, but in the end, it was up to me to change myself for once and stop listening to the dark consciousness in my head telling me I'm a good-for-nothing nobody who will be isolated from society forever.

I blamed my older brother a lot for this as he was the one I used to look up to when I was young and I lost a friend whom I missed because of him. I think that's why I became a bully in school after losing her. I put up my barriers after that, shut the door to him for good, promised myself for as long as I don't see her, I want nothing to do with him and that he doesn't exist in my life.

But, at the end of the day, there was no one to blame for the position I put myself into. I was so hot and bothered wanting so many answers at once that I couldn't feel myself inside or outside and became a ghost along with all the manipulative effects from medications. I may have still been breathing, but I couldn't sense anything for instance. I often was called by my name in town or someone would beep the horn at me and I'd hear them perfectly. But, at the same time, I'd say to myself they're hardly calling me; who wants anything to do with me, and then that would confuse me, and I wouldn't even check.

I used to look at the homeless people and wonder if I was going down that path even though I was at home. I always saw myself as the outsider and I wondered if those people were on the streets for that reason too because some of the most intelligent people can end up homeless and that's when you should question the world we're living in today. Why do they end up in the gutter and I think it's because they know so much and can see so far ahead that it frightens them and stops them from wanting to be part of society. They turn to a simple life with nothing to lose and begin to drink or do drugs like tortured artists trying to shut down their creative side. That just leads to being homeless, which to some, after so long becomes normal, but the depression gets so worse after the drink, which is why I never drank while I had it because I knew I would definitely be dead now. So that's why my mind was way too overactive because I had nothing to numb it until I was out of work for nearly a year and finally began to do art again.

That's what slowly began to ease the pain bit by bit. Exercising art and meeting others who were into art was what I slowly tried to create. A new me gradually came out of it, and here I'll describe how bad my mental health was.

I used to say the most negative things to myself such as if I have a bad day today, maybe tomorrow will be a little better and it was the same with the seizures and anxiety and that used to stabilize things out for a while. This was positive enough at the start until I got into this phase of looking at positive words of the English alphabet. Dog, devil, life was the most common ones of all and then began to say them backward, which are god, lived, evil□and this used to fascinate me into an overactive consciousness from negative thinking, not aware that I was the only person locked into my consciousness who was thinking this way.

I thought I was ahead of others and that I cracked a new code or something, thinking like this where I was isolating myself even more than before and I couldn't think straight at all. I began to give every word a different meaning as if it was my language. I once asked my mother what does stress means? When I was there myself for the last few years experiencing it and she just looked at me as if I should know, but I didn't and also didn't even understand the word 'depression' at that time from too much isolation and overthinking. My consciousness was elsewhere.

What I did achieve going through this is not drinking or doing drugs, I do and still, believe that anyone drinking who suffers from depression will only make things more difficult to recover and the longer you accept the abuse you give yourself, the longer it will go on and become worse. Alcohol may relieve stress, but here in Ireland we drink way too much and make a mess of our lives from alcohol, which some may forget, is an actual anti-depressant too. It can only relieve stress for so long until people get hooked on it and waste themselves away from others. Over 1000 lives are taken each year from this drug that's legal to use while over 600 plus are taken from prescription drugs that are legal and supposed to make us better which adds up to more people than die on our roads that we never hear the end of.

I've no sympathy for people who won't help themselves when they know they can do it, but I do for people who isolate themselves and don't know their way out. The population in our country is small compared to others; some of us just drink ourselves away, gradually that becomes our lifestyle and we find it amusing. I like the odd drink now and then, but I am not spending every cent I have on it and destroying my insides that will never be able to fully recover. If we can't care for ourselves, no one else is there to care for us. Live a little, look forward, and lead the way to where your destination is, and don't give up. Hope for the better, and if you stay afloat, one day your hope will come when you least expect it.

Also, in today's world due to our levels of ignorance, we have corruption with corporations who are up to all sorts when in 2012, (Glaxo Smith Kline) one of the world's largest pharmaceutical companies admitted to promoting Paxil and Wellbutrin for unapproved uses. This included the treatment of children and adolescents. This, in turn, is called an off-label practice is known as off-label marketing along with many other global players that put profit before lives.

PSYCHIATRY

My first appointment with counseling was with a psychologist in Cork City for my behavior problems after I had finished school to see why I was behaving the way I was. They were going to try to structure my behavior — that was only from frustration from having nobody listen or understand me for a few years now — and see the faults to be able to fix them along with all the side effects from medications while I was still developing.

But now, when I look back, it's quite obvious why I was simply behaving the way I was. I had turned sour towards everyone and everything that let me down. I also became frustrated when I saw other people doing simple things I was restricted from doing due to my condition. But, I was well able to do them all, and every time I stepped out of line doing little things I was going to do anyway, I was being told not to do that because it was too dangerous or I could have a seizure. These are negative statements as could and might are two different words.

So, if anything, I was being led into a negative outlook when all I wanted to do were simple things I knew I was well capable of doing anyway from a very young age like climbing trees, cycling, and swimming. I couldn't stand knowing that people were worried about me. I still can't to this day because I'm my person like everyone else is. I have my ambition to create my statistics and work strategies in life, to succeed in certain things I can do. Most of all, I have the dream to be fully healthy. I've known since I was a child that I'm destined to be successful at something in this world like everyone else is, and my way of thinking will take me there rather than going the same way as everyone else, especially when I'm not living the same way as them.

At the end of the day, we all have our destiny if we want to go our way or not and some of us manage to feel fulfilled while some of us don't. Maybe because I was my person, I always felt like the outsider who never fit in anyway. So, I had to build my life path and create my destination because I always went with my instincts from an early age, no matter what bumps or twists were in the way because it felt right, not because it sounded right when I thought about it.

One particular time, I was sour towards my dad as he was always keeping an eye on me and would make sure that I was corrected if I did something wrong just like any parent would. But I hated being corrected as I felt I had enough to deal with personally and was frustrated due to the things I wasn't allowed to do, so sometimes, I refused to be corrected because I was not a slave, I was human. Due to all these corrections, I knew it would be this atmosphere I would be living in for quite a while through childhood. I became busier thinking how I was going to find a way to keep everyone happy rather than having to listen to them worry so much and think I was not able to do other things that they were. The more they worried, the sourer I got and the more I felt the guilt due to being sick and refusing to be controlled by them for my safety.

But his way of rearing a good kid was letting them know who is boss and who calls the shots, and if something needed to be said, it would be by him. Due to what I had, I was going to be treated differently, and if I acted out of control, I would be treated even more differently. But I felt the only difference was that I got seizures often but the medications were much worse than them, nothing else. It was the same as somebody deciding to get drunk once a week and linking themselves to a different consciousness for that short space of time till they become sober again. I was angrier each time I was corrected because I was well able to do things that I was restricted from doing like cycling or swimming. But, I didn't understand that I also had to learn that I couldn't always have what I wanted at the same time, even if I was able to do things I was not supposed to do.

One time, I told the psychologist out of frustration that I either got a smack or I was sent to my room or I was told that the guards were coming to take me away. My dad would simply throw me into my room and make sure I learned what was right from wrong even though I knew what was right from wrong. But, my head was never still and the effects of drugs I was taking were never understood. I wasn't going to live a silent life and say nothing about things that were happening to me.

But when I grew up a little and saw how people work with each other when they grow up, I used to tell nobody anything anymore so they wouldn't feed on the early trauma I had experienced. He was making a point, whether I liked it or not, by disciplining me. He was not going to let me get my way like no one can in this world anyway, so him being right and me refusing to be controlled fully by him and the illness began to create distance between us as the years went on, with all the ignorance and drama that it created. All I wanted to do was find a way out of the home to just feel free again. But, he never gave up on rearing us all the way he knew was right because I would have become more confused if I finally got my way and would have acted upon something else if he did let me get my way, wondering all the while what all the fuss was about in the first all those years.

In some ways, you could say that I was an attention seeker looking for answers too early about what's wrong with me that I couldn't control or why I couldn't be left to do simple things when I was perfectly capable of doing them but had no idea about law, politics, or the constitution. That just became more confusing as life went on, but my parents did everything they could to help me out of this messy anxiety. Back then, Ireland's culture's demand regarding how to live was still very strong to earn your place, and I lost all interest in fitting in with society after realizing the restrictions I was supposed to live up to rather than the things I was not allowed do in general.

I feel I've always been ruled by my emotions, and whatever I feel towards something is the strength I drive towards, however big or small it is. See, all this disabled structure was shattered in me due to feeling left out and being treated differently in the first place. This kept me far from satisfied from an early age, and I felt cursed and kept searching for an answer to how I can do everything I needed without annoying someone else to get it. The fact is if I knew how to move out of home at that time, I would have given it a go and worked my way up any ladder. Fair enough, I accepted the fact that I had a condition, and no matter what, I had to deal with it; whether everyone turned against me or not. I still had to put up with that whatever the case, until I found a way out of it.

My way of standing up to the psychologists here and not being led by doctors — who were treated as gods — was to do everything that I was told not to do, to prove to myself that I'm not the person in the corner to be controlled by whoever these people think they are, and I do have feelings. The system in which people like me get told to hide in the corner away from society till they're better was something I began to give the two fingers to from the start because if that's the case, we are all disabled with separate faults and should all go and hide in our corners. There was no way I was ever going to be looked down on as an issue or a big problem, so every time I was treated like that or felt I was, I acted up in self-defense.

The disabled are not criminals; like the kids in Third World countries — starving or infected — are not. They're living in the real world with higher challenges than others to get over and could live a practical, normal life without any hesitation if they were left alone in the right system. I became sourer, the less I was being listened to. I knew it was hard work, but it was because I was telling the truth about everything — like what the medications were doing to my body and Gerard being frustrated and getting away with it time after time — and again, nobody was listening. This was because the American dream was starting and everyone was following it even though it was a new dream while I lived in the reality of corporate greed, so a gap was soon created between me and society.

I wasn't going to the corner acting all 'poor me', and I wasn't going to be allowed to have my way either. So, all I wanted was an identity and to show people I may not be perfect but it's me that lives with this condition and it's my system that's swallowing these medications every day, which were not solving the problem. I just wanted to be understood, but I wasn't. So my anger grew month after month, year after year, especially through my teens and I just stopped explaining myself to my family anymore and just went completely quiet as nothing positive was happening, no matter how hard I tried to explain and I was never believed.

I became extremely out of balance towards them. I was very much in mode to myself, but of course, that was in my little sour world of consciousness that was growing with rage from the frustration of the effects that I was feeling. I was sliding into my first experience of depression at this time, slowly but surely. A huge volume of thoughts went through my head each day on how I wanted to end my life as I couldn't find anything or anyone that was able to understand me and wanted more than anything not to be part of this controlled identity.

It amazes me how I'm still here today when I look back, I had a completely overactive mind that I couldn't compare with anyone back then. The fact that everyone else was on similar levels, relating themselves to each other, I could do no right or be understood. On top of that, I had an overactive imagination full of frustration, growing towards feeling uncontrollably resentful about how to get out of the mess I was in.

I think I'm a natural thinker anyway, in how everything works in this world, and have always aimed as high as I could imagine, to try and make it all real. So I grew more and more frustrated due to the position I was in. My acting out became more frequent, the fewer people that understood me, the more tortured I felt.

Shortly after that, to some extent, the negativity just took over and created much anxiety and little satisfaction with anything anymore. I was fifteen and had left school due to the failure of the system with people with my condition. The vice-principal in Dun Lock Secondary School said to my mother, "He needs psychological help" and "do not bring him back since he has lost his temper too many times".

So, after that incident which I did not start, my mum rang a local minister and met him for coffee and explained the anger I had been expressing. He booked a bed for me in Dublin psychiatric ward to get help for my anger problems as I was probably fit to damage someone with the rage in me at that age from all this frustration. My parents were worried about how angry I used to get so they sent me to Dublin psychiatric ward two weeks after leaving Dun Lock School.

The fact is that I may have been listened to in this place by them, but I still wasn't understood by anyone who was working in the system as they looked more educated by their ego than their positions. However, I was understood more by the other people in there for different treatments. The staff in there was asking me questions as if I knew what's right from wrong. At the end of the day, I was the one who was looking for answers in the system they were making a living off that people like me, who are medicated, pay for.

I understood they needed my help for what was wrong with me, but there's only so much question you can take before your expectations begin to inflate with false solutions, and if it doesn't happen, then that says the system they were working with has failed miserably. What was in it for me? Nothing. Plenty of questions and time but no concrete answers. So can you blame me for the way I was acting compared to the way I was being treated, over and over?

So, I felt more lost in myself every time I was misunderstood because I was not lying about anything I was asked. Again, they just didn't have what I did or understood the effects I was trying to tell them about the medications. They just studied social care or psychology but never had any mental issues in the real world themselves. They didn't have the tools to understand my situation or some other people's either, and I was living with real problems in the real world, which are two different situations to them working in a system. So I was just again annoyed with the system and that anyone could just come by and enter the field as long as they're intelligent enough, with some degree in college paid by the massive corporation again. Every time I showed how annoyed I was about being revenue for the system, I was classified as an issue. It never gave me more motivation or any confidence when other people gave me a compliment for going through all this because I was not out there to make them happy.

I had to show them that while not everyone succeeds in school, some that leave can still aim high due to the way their consciousness is wired with the way the world's growing.

But, in the real world, it's yourself that you need to make happy first and not others, as too many are frightened of screwing up in front of others. They produce in themselves a comfort zone to the only aim to certain levels of success which simply regulates their character and outlook and pretty much grounds them for the rest of their days. In Dublin Psychiatric Centre, shortly after leaving school, I got on with all the others well with similar circumstances in their lives and was thrilled to finally meet people who understood me better than others I knew due to their conditions.

I remember a certain guy in there who gave me a wake-up call due to his condition as he had two disabilities, which I won't name, but had also drifted into depression from the isolation they gave him. So I told him my situation, and we shared each other's views of the health system. He showed me the music he listens to, which was R.E.M. "Everybody Hurts" was one of his favourites, and I turned around and said, "Do you not think that would kind of make you feel more isolated because it is not very uplifting and the frame of consciousness you're already in?"

He said, "You're right, but it keeps me level, knowing where I stand."

I shook my head and said, "Well, if that's your music now, you'll be into heavy metal in no time with the frustration you'll put yourself through." He nodded his head and laughed. Then, he asked if I'd bring him outside since he couldn't walk at the time. I said, "I thought we are not allowed outside in here," and he said, "You're allowed to go outside for half an hour if you want." So, I brought him out, pushed him around, and on the way back to the ward, he lashed out, and I said, "What's wrong with you?" and he said, "I'm sick of it," and told me to stop pushing him and leave him alone.

So, I didn't understand his reaction that he was expressing his loneliness and said, "What did I do?" and he said, "Go away and leave me alone," and lashed out at me, smacking me and taking my hands off the chair. So, I smacked him back and then went back to my bed and began smacking my bed since I had done nothing wrong.

As soon as I was seen doing this, the nurses came over to me along with security and took me upstairs to a room where I was locked into for the night with me only wearing a pair of jeans. I wasn't even allowed to keep my shoes or T-shirt in case I tried to hang myself even though there was no object around the ceiling I could have done that with. I thought this was dramatic altogether.

I thought that was extreme for someone who started punching a bed and had not killed anyone or been labeled with any mental disorder, but I suppose I just wasn't in the right frame of consciousness back then to control my anger each time I lashed out and acted, only too frequently. But, the cause was of course never listened to, and they had to look out for the rest of the people in the ward at the time who I wouldn't have touched but couldn't be trusted for that. So, the next day I was back in the ward and was very calm but very annoyed with the system too, but I got rid of plenty of anger that night lashing out with whatever rage that was left in me, but I wasn't standing for people's abuse either whatever way I was or labeled as. I know I was way out of control and exhausted from been ignored for so long and not understood for that matter.

So, shortly after coming back to the ward, I went to meet the psychiatrists the next day as that was the normal routine every morning to see how each person's getting on in there. I was fit to shout at them as they could see I was far from scared of them all looking at them sit down taking down notes of people's actions and looking all smart and fancy. I may have only been fifteen, but I had a lot of experience in the real world too. I was thinking the way things work in there was their fault never knowing who funded it or anything like that.

The fact is I was always searching for answers that they just never answered, and I was always the one being asked questions and was tired of answering them and keeping them in a job. He looked at me and asked "Do you find any help here?" and I said to be honest only people who understand me here are the other patients; the people who work here are not any help and many patients end up coming back after relapsing.

Then, he said this is not the place for you and sent me back to my room to pack my bags and I said to myself, "You got that right. I didn't care and just walked out of there with more disappointment and said to myself, "I was glad to be out."

So, my parents came up after I spent nearly a week in there and I said my goodbyes to all the other patients in there and walked out to the car and my mum said to me before I got into the car, "Did you learn anything in there?"

I nodded yes, and she replied, "Are you going to calm down so and start behaving?"

I just nodded again and in my consciousness and began to get a little frustrated as I was not a little child anymore, but she was probably thinking he will be treated well when he earns it or whatever else. But, I'd enough on my mind to go earning respect or try to please others now, but she is my mother, so I looked at her and said thanks for coming up, and my dad put the bags into the back. We drove home. I said to myself on the way back, I should for once listen to her and just go along with her.

So, I returned home, and as far as I can remember, I think I was okay for a few months or so knowing now that there are others in my situation around, and hoped to keep in contact with them. But, as far as technology came then, it was not that simple to keep friends who lived up the country, which today to me is only a click away due to the speed society has taken with technology since. So, I was at home in Saleen keeping to myself washing cars for people and cycling around doing people's windows and gardens to make some money until one day my younger brother saw me play his friend's computer as I had asked his friend Kevin if it was okay and he let me use it.

Then, my brother Patrick wanted money off me for playing it. I said no, and he asked again, "Give me money for playing it," and I turned to him and said, "It's not yours." He then grabbed the joystick off me. I took it back and told him to go away, and he went for it again, so I lost my temper, thumping him like crazy on the head.

My mum heard us and came in and had to drag me off him at this point. And I just ran away as I just couldn't be forced to go into detail about what just happened and it wasn't as if anyone was going to listen anyway as I didn't start it but did manage to finish it. So, I began to feel sour again realizing no matter what I will always be alone in this and went down to Lemybrien to a friend and told him the situation that my mother had called the guards and was going to lock me up again. He said you're too young☐they can't lock you up for anything! My anxiety had taken over already after being in Dublin psychiatric center was enough drama because my mum had called the guards as soon as I left. Then, I walked over to a lake there, and for the first time, I started to seriously think if I'd be better off dead away from family and let them get on with their own lives well away from me.

I didn't see this going anywhere now and certainly didn't feel wanted there or part of them, so I became so interested in ending my life that it became a stable and numb feeling at the same time. I realized if all comes to bad, everything can end at once, and I can just kill myself.

So, by thinking like that, the loneliness and sourness began to ease a little, and the consciousness wasn't in overdrive as usual. So, I began to plan everything out from scratch and was enjoying the fact that for once, I was back in control of a plan I had because it could change everything not realizing what I would have left behind, but what I didn't seem to realize is that it could also end everything for good at the same time which was quite scary.

When I look back, that thought had never come to my mind before then. My behavior then began to change depending on who I was with as I was not one of those who forgave and forget individuals that quick either, so at home, I was still annoyed because I hated living at home anyway growing up where I just didn't feel any bit of comfort or understanding. But, with my friends, it varied depending on how close I was with them, and I did have a few close ones who never would go spreading my issues around or feed on the situations I was in as my mum was too much of a worrier. I could never tell her anything as I felt she would have no problem telling her friends and not see anything wrong with it either, which I did completely see a lot wrong with it, so from there on, I began to drift away from home and closer to my friends. The closer, the better.

As I was a constant thinker of a better way to do things, I spent a lot of time alone planning to kill myself in many different ways and many different places; and I told no one, not even my closest friends for a long time. This plan was like my new identity to me saying that I own this and no one's going to know about it if I manage to do it. It was a bit like finally having a bit of dignity to myself after searching for years because everyone knew my business, and that alone made my stomach turn as I believed not all but many only wanted to see someone worse off than themselves but became good at been naive anyway.

I only used to tell people certain things to keep them as certain loyal friends. I'm like that because I'm quite a sensitive person who can only open up certain areas of myself to certain people. If I let someone know all of me, then they're close, so in the end, I told Shiv who I met in hospital many years before when I was young, and Nigel who I knew very well too.

Shiv would urge me to stop thinking like that or she will tell my parents and Nigel told me he feels like doing the same sometimes but doesn't think he would ever do such a thing. I went for regular check-ups every few months to Cork Medical Centre since I was a child.

One time when I was about eighteen, I was fed up with medications and even more fed up nobody was listening to the abuse they were causing. It felt as if they had more of a chance of killing me with the effects than stopping me from ever have seizures. They created horrible emotional manipulation to my body that people can't see but you can feel, and the more I was on them the harder the effects became, I found I was living to survive over time. Seizures were still frequent if not worse, and I told Dr. O' Donovan who was my doctor in Cork Medical till I was eighteen how I was feeling, which was ending my life, and he asked me to draw a horse to see if I was going insane. I refused to with the stubbornness of been misunderstood again because they say if you're going insane, your creativity fades.

But, mine was far from faded so I looked at him as if I saw him with two heads because my mind was perfectly fine just far from stable, but I was frustrated from people's ignorance again. Ignore-ance□the word itself even explains how many problems it can cause, and the more important people feel☐ego☐ the more ignore-ant they can become, and I felt he was one of them after asking such a stupid question.

Then he asked me if I would go to Cork psychiatric center for treatment, and at this point, it was either help or become more suicidal, so I asked what kind of people go there and what would it do for me?

Hoping that it would not link to what happened in Dublin Psychiatric Centre, which was a waste of time. He said people in your condition who are depressed or are in worse conditions go there normally for a week or two to seek help and balance out their condition, and if you don't like it, you won`t have to stay there cause you're now an adult and not forced to go. So, I was also closer to home and I could sign out if it did not agree with me so I went in there later that evening.

When I went in there, it was like a youth jail, which reminded me of the room I was put into in Dublin for losing my temper. I was checked in and told to strip all my clothes and belongings off, and everything was taken off me. I was given these very light pajamas that could have been considered as cloth rather than cotton as the material was so weak in it that if you tried anything with it, it would tear instantly.

I felt out of it in there and even worse felt very degraded and cheap, and they were putting a lot of people to sleep by giving them drugs every few hours in there explaining to me when I asked that it's just something to make them relax. Most were becoming like zombies in there. It wasn't my place to be at all and I thanked God I could sign myself out of such a place where before that was never possible depending on your condition. But, I needed to see it for myself to realize that I was not on the right path the way I was thinking and behaving, and this place would have made me a lot worse. If anything, similar to last time, it was the description of seeing the other patients in there who were in worse situations already after cutting themselves or had been raped is that gave me a big eye-opener. I saw that places like that if anything can slow down a lot of people's mobility and life structure for a very long time as the more they spend in there, the more they believe something bigger is wrong with them and must start to value life more whatever is going on.

The support is not well given in these places either. I felt while I was in there that the structure of running these places was very old and wrong due to the world's population now growing at one billion each decade and declining less at this stage. This tells that these places will have more and more people going to them, and the faults of the system will keep occurring unless they change strategies in helping rather than mass medicating.

We all get tensed and pressured into things we don't particularly like or fit into through our lives. But, I think the world should be run and structured by population for everyone to feel someway driven to succeed same way a business is by finance but for the right reasons and not the massive powerful psychotic ways by psychotic people who should be put into these places for at least a year or two.

Because we're all peer pressured and drawn to different measures and statistics that we all want different things at separate stages of our lives. To keep the world in a system, we have to work by population and needs to strengthen structure into systems for the people rather than elites as independence was fought by people for the people and not by elites for elites. More and more people want different things in life and will get their satisfaction in it whatever needs have to be met same as a determined person wants to make their goals a reality. So, nearly a year later, after I had signed myself out of Cork Psychiatric Centre only after been there a few days. I had continued to go downhill with emotional stress during the times of going for so many separate tests to cork hospital too at this time. My whole life of lessons was literally all conceived into one at this time and things were going downhill as I got deeply depressed and still felt like ending my life.

I still said to myself, Why come this far and then end it, so I was put on Cipramil an (anti-depressant), which gave me a little boost as time went on, and they then put me into another psychiatric unit in cork which was attached to the hospital I always stayed in growing up and put the dosage up.

Again with little confidence in these places, I was fed up of been sent to them and was talking to all the others in there who were a lot worse off again and wondered how in god's name did I end up in here and what benefit is it doing for the others either? I began questioning myself, where exactly should I be? And as a result of feeling little confidence as usual in such places and deeper depression, putting the dosage up for depression made me worse and I refused to eat and talk and just felt drained and completely out of touch in some way like a zombie. Then I rang my mum and said this place is a joke and, "I'm signing out, I don't belong in here at all!"

Every time I've done such things it was very like a relapse expect it made me stronger in many ways rather than playing the victim in the system. She didn't know what to say, and my dad rang back an hour later telling me to stay in there until the doctors tell me you're okay to go. I said, "No, this place isn't for me, I've been in these places too many times." So, he replied, "Okay, I don't know what to say but if you're sure then it`s up to you." So, I packed my bags and signed out, and walked out that evening.

On top of that, I also stopped taking the anti-depressants slowly coming off on them and felt much better than I did on them. However, a week later the relapse returned since the chemicals were been released from my system. So, I expected this to happen and knew it was going to be bad, and again at this time I wanted to slit my throat, which lasted a whole week, and I was sweating with thoughts of suicide.

But, I stayed off them knowing it was only the chemicals leaving my body. But, all I wanted was to be understood more than anything about the psychotic industry, if only someone could agree with me to show me I'm not going insane like I felt I was and not have people tell me they don't know what to say.

So, I was again frustrated and lost but it was obvious I was going to feel lost if nobody similar was around in my situation and question the whole system so I could interact and heal with them. It wasn't my mum's fault that I felt I couldn't open up to her or describe what I felt was wrong with me cause I didn't even fully know at the time myself how bad I was, so she couldn't understand me since I couldn't fully understand myself. It's the way I felt about myself and even misunderstood myself at times, but I was always up for a new challenge that was possible to help me out of the situations I was in. It's why I think I had no problem going into these places first. That was the third and final time I was in these places, and I met this other girl in there who was cutting herself to release pain from inside. That's why people cut themselves, to feel human and normal again and release the pain they feel. These units should be separate rooms for separate conditions the fact so many are in there for completely different reasons altogether and one person in there might be twenty times worse than another scaring the person who is not as bad to run out of the place.

The goal for most people with a mental health problem I think is simply a new atmosphere to live in a new consciousness and higher spirit than they are currently living in. People are the fastest way of finding such things rather than mass-medicating them with lethal drugs because people are meant to be interacting with each other and helping each other out with community spirit and so on. And over 500,000 people are killed from psychiatric drugs every year in the western world alone which adds up to Kazakhstan's whole population in about 36 years with the majority of these deaths been over 65 years of age and not one war out there to take down such psychotic profit war on health. So, there must be some serious mental health problems with people who retire to be medicated like that yet they have most of the money made too. So, what it says to me is how fast psychotic greed can de-populate.

Escaping pain

My way of escaping from all the reality of everyday living and all the built-up pressure and depression from everything never had anything to do with drinking alcohol or taking any type of drugs as the medications I was on legally were causing enough problems.

I could see past all that behavior knowing that if there was any way of me been cured someday, the effects of alcohol or drugs will still be there. I didn't want to ever be going around with a paranoid mind slowly reacting to most everyday things when I already had to grow up with something I was not able to control.

Drugs can do no more than kill all the cells in your brain, which is why you have that high that you enjoy but take little notice of what the effect will do in the long run and also have to realize there always comes a low with a high same as a bust after a boom bubble. I had a wise idea already from the abuse the medications had caused me to go through while I was developing but also was trying to find any way to get off them too.

But, I had this threat that my mother had built into me that if I do go off them I could or will die, which is why I had to stay on them after trying it once before and ending up having a grand mal seizure over a week later cause I came right off them rather than slowly. That threat annoyed me continually, so if I was to become the self-pitying individual, rather than the self-destructive type. Then, of course, I would have drunk myself to death with alcohol and taken all the drugs that were possible at the time, which is a fact.

So, sometimes it makes me wonder if someone was watching over me as I always did feel one of my grandfathers close to me that I never even remember meeting. And could not explain how I knew it was him protecting me much of the time. So I took a different route, and from the age of seventeen to twenty-three, I went on the road around Ireland.

Since I wasn't allowed to drive with epilepsy, I did it by bus and train, each weekend after work, I would pick a place out of the blue and just go there. It used to open my senses and give me a sense of freedom for just a tiny period. It also showed me how the real world is and what kind of things people get up to and what length some would go to just to survive in separate parts of the country and economy.

It made me realize no matter how sick I am or how bad I get, I was never going to neglect myself into a black hole and fade myself away from society as a loner or waste of space whatever the dangers and situations are because of having temporal lobe epilepsy. It's not that I even wanted to be in society because I never did and don't much of the time like many. I've seen the real world for a long time.

So, after work each Friday, I used to pack my bag, say bye to my mum when I lived at home hoping she won't start worrying, and my friends when I moved out of home and race to the bus station in Cork to pick a county on where to go for the weekend. I would go there straightaway without hesitation on where to stay and had no plans on what to do when I got there. I knew the travel system someway from now from working with my dad for so long, traveling around the country analyzing systems on the roads.

I guessed that hostels, bed and breakfasts, and hotels will always be options open wherever I go as it was very rare I'd go to the countryside unless I was more closed and in need to open up. Most of the time it was Dublin I went to since it had a straight route from Cork every two hours and was pretty easy to find a place to stay since it was the capital with some places open twenty-four hours a day. The fact everything would be open late and the busier the better as nobody wants to know your business when life's too busy but that's not good for a relationship of course.

So, it just made more sense to go there in the end, and I loved sitting in the bus at night passing through the towns full of lights and especially seen them coming towards the towns and cities. This used to fascinate me with all the effects from the shadows and created a structure of a built town or city lit up like a map of lights. This was an effect I used to try and use in the art I do too as it shows the system of the city or town in place.

I've always had a fascination with maps from a very young age and still do to this day as I believe they tell the structure and dominance of how fast our industrialized world has been created and how fast we have linked to each other's nations that lead to global culture in my eyes. This routine of going to Dublin was going on for about a year, my first departure at seventeen was Waterford city since I knew my dad worked down there a lot and I was renting a place in cork where I could go there anytime from as it passed the road to there.

So, I became bored one weekend and decided to go with Waterford only two hours away by bus. So, I hopped on one Saturday morning and went there, and was already down there a few times with my dad. So, I knew my way around there a little, and as soon as I got off the bus, I went across the road to a bed and breakfast and got myself a bedroom, which was right on the key of Waterford city which is also the oldest city in Ireland too, so again I was happy as long as I could look at the lights at night flicking away in the river that always amused me for some reason or another. So, I went out that night and wandered around the city amused with how elaborate a small city can be with many different atmospheres in many different public houses and the fact I didn't drink alcohol I saw so much more realistic on how people act in their spare time after a few drinks.

That same night, I learned more about peer pressure than any other time as I was in a bar drinking a Coke and put mon-ey up on the pool table for the next game, and as soon as my turn came up, I got beaten. The guy that I was playing against was around thirty, and he said whoever wins buys a drink, and that was fine with me. So, I won, and he asked what am I drinking, and I said, "Coke." He asked, "Why Coke?"

I told him, "I don't drink alcohol." He asked, "Why not?" I replied, "I just don't as I've never touched it and don't see the point when I see what it does to people."

Then, he paused for a bit and looked around the pub shaking his head, and finally bought me a Coke, but then he tried to urge me to taste his drink which was Jack Daniels and coke. He was putting it up to my mouth and telling me to taste it and I said "I'm not interested, don't even bother!"

Then, I asked what does he do, and he said he was a chef at Cronin's and I said, "Are you on about the hotel across from the bridge?"

And he said yes he had just been laid off recently, and I asked about his family to which he replied he had and has broken up with them too, so I assumed that this is just what life's going to be all about, full of problems. Then a few minutes later,

I said to him, "I'm heading away," and he asked where I'm staying. I said, "Down by the bridge in a bed and breakfast," and he said he will walk with me. I said, "It's okay," but he said, "Come on, I'll walk down." So, he walked with me and came into the bar where I was staying above and ordered a drink for him and me. I flopped it and said "I must go, I'm wrecked," and little did he know I might get a seizure if I don't sleep as I never told him I had epilepsy but was going to get one or two in a week anyway. Then I said, "Where are you staying?" as I didn't think he had anywhere, and he said, "I'm not sure yet," and I said, "I've got a bed upstairs as I'm in a twin room, you can stay there."

His face dropped with shame, a seventeen-year-old saying this to a guy nearly twice his age and he said thanks. He stayed that night and went off the next morning, A few hours later, I packed my bags and went off home for another week's work. A few weeks later, I went to Waterford again but stayed somewhere different as I was on my holidays and had more time off, so I spent one night in a flat. It cost me only eighty pounds at the time, but I had a great time since it was the first time I came across satellite TV and a balcony by the water and a public phone all in one.

So, I went off for a walk around eleven p.m. in Waterford by the key, and this was the first time I came across prostitution when I saw a woman dressed with hardly anything on and cars driving up and she just hoped in.

It was the only time I saw it in Waterford right across from the bus station that was beside the train station at the time. Apart from that, I once asked the taxi driver there, "Where do they get off doing this to themselves never knowing they had to make a living in some way."

 I thought I was bad enough with what I had and they seem to have perfect health, but I never knew anything about any mental health issue and what addictions some people can have yet either or personal and financial circumstances that could lead to something like that, which made me very narrow-minded about it at the time. The taxi driver was telling me that there usually in the pubs now rather than the streets and I again just shook my head with confusion. The next morning, I went home on the bus back to Cork wondering if this carries on in Cork city too as cork is the second biggest after Dublin? So a few weeks later I went to Cork with a few friends and told them about what I saw in Waterford.

They said they're in Cork too, and I said, "Where?"

They replied they're down by the keys too, so I pretty much got the idea the keys were their location by now. I said, "How long have these things being going on."

He replied, "Years, people do it mainly to make a living or feed a habit."

I said, "Yes, I pretty much got that idea in Waterford. I just think it's sad to see people sell themselves so easily and worse that people enjoy using each other to fill an urge here and there?"

This began to interest me to try and establish a situation away from it. So, one day after I found where they were I walked up to one in Cork and asked, "Why are you here?"

She said, "Are you interested or not?" I shook my head saying "No, just want to know why you here like this."

She told me where to go, so I took a twenty-pound note out and said "Here, take that, but I'm just wondering why people do these things."

She said she was kicked out of home by her dad and has no way of finding herself and doesn't want to go home anyway.

I tapped her on the shoulder and said, "I'm sorry!" This girl must have been only eighteen at the most. Then I went home and began to write how I felt about these ongoing situations.

The next Friday, I went to Limerick since it was another city I had never been to, and I got the bus from Cork and got off in Limerick and booked a bed and breakfast. Limerick was fairly big to me at this time compared to Waterford, so I said I better be extra safe here and ignored most people. So, after I booked in, I walked around Limerick and wondered if prostitution was also here like it was in Waterford and cork. I couldn't see any of it, and I walked over to the bridges and around the keys and turned back towards the city and saw a pub that was jam-packed with college students.

I went in and people were looking for trouble around and stared at me once or twice, and one particular person put his cigarettes out on my new top after I was only there about ten minutes. I took the top off and took his jacket that was beside him on the chair, and stood on it. I said to him, "What are you going to do now?"

He grabbed his jacket off the floor staring at me and went back to his mates. I walked away then looking for somewhere else to browse but decided to head back to the bed and breakfast as I had enough of Limerick already since it had the name stab city with a crime rate the same as Dublin even though it has not even ten percent of Dublin's population.

As I was walking back, a guy behind me asked for the time, and I said I don't know. His reply was, "Yes, what do you know? In a drunken state."

I turned around and said, "Sorry?" He smiled and said nothing back. I couldn't wait to get away from Limerick and said to myself, This is a place I won't miss much. So a few weeks later, I went back to

Waterford on a mission to see if I'd see anything new in Waterford and the fact the people were a lot more kind there too similar to cork.

The next day after been there for the night, I decided to go away further since it was a really warm day so I packed my bags up. I walked to the bus station in Waterford, and since it was an early Saturday morning, I said, "I'll try Dublin for the first time knowing well it was much bigger than Cork from seen it on the TV all the time, And I should be even more careful up there than I was in Limerick."

So, I went on the bus and got all the money I had, which I forgot to do in Limerick, and put it under my sock in case I was robbed. A few hours later when I got there I was shocked coming into the city seen lights everywhere and taking over twenty minutes to even get to the city center and was also surprised with how quick the time goes and said to myself, This place is very big. So, I got off the bus at Busarus in Dub-lin city center and began to wander around for a place to stay, so I took a long walk up Gardeners Street until it became too quiet and walked back down and got to the closest hostel to the bus station.

I paid up for two nights and went away walking around the city for hours again. I was trying to figure out how these places work and the illusion and collective consciousness that Orcastrates demand for everything engineering the city to become bigger and bigger. As I got answers from a taxi driver in

Waterford, I learned that if you want to know anything, ask the taxi drivers since they know the cities they drive in inside out!

So, I hailed down a taxi and said, "Where does everyone go out here?" He asked, "What sort of place are you looking for?"

I told him just somewhere to hang out that's busy with little dress codes. He said Temple Bar has everything but some have a dress code, so I said, "What about somewhere to just relax with some rock music."

He said (the Kingston rock) so he took me there just over five minutes away. I showed them my ID as I had just turned eighteen and wasn't drinking anyway, so I went down the stairs and in to the bar and got a Coke. It was so much like the rock bar in cork where everyone is everyone without the no drama, or false commercial behavior. It was those places I began to grow to like more. Some of the most down-to-earth people can be found in these public houses that are known to higher class people as nobodies, which I think is truly wrong to class all the people going to these places as that type because of what they wear or listen to!

I went there often each time I went to Dublin and one time I had a seizure in there, felt it come on, and said to myself Oh shit! I hope they don't think I'm on drugs," while I was having the 'aura'.

I knew if I spoke out loud, I would have it right away, so I sat there hoping it would ease and hopefully not have one. If so, I would head back to the hostel straight away especially with Dublin city being new to me. But, I had a seizure and the security was fine and knew what was wrong with me, which was very surprising to me because each time this happened in other parts of the country, they misunderstood the problem thinking I was on drugs or too drunk from alcohol and threw me out the door on to the streets. But, in Dublin, they took care of me as I was more or less expecting to be thrown out on the street again like I was in cork many times. They knew the problem and waited for me to come around and asked where I was staying. I eventually could pronounce Gardeners Street as it was only around the corner from the bus station, and it's where I always stayed.

So, the security called me a taxi to drop me back, and I thanked them saying, "Sorry for the hassle but just because I have this problem, I can't lock myself indoors," and they said, "Don't worry about it, do what you like."

I smiled and said to myself, Damn right, I will.

Weeks went by, then months went by, and I said to myself, Why not go abroad for a change?

I packed my bag and said I'll try hitchhiking to London which is about 450km from cork but it's the main road only for the ferry on the way across the water, so not having a clue where I'll stay again or the next place I could end up having a seizure I just started it. Because once I was active, I wasn't as negative towards anything and I was much calmer. So, off I went hitching in cork aiming for Rosslare harbor also not knowing if I'd even make the ferry, so I got as far as Waterford City. It was lashing out of the heavens and I said the hell with it as a storm had started. I said, "I'll stay there tonight."

Wherever I stayed had to be on a street and by the window as all the lights been lit up at night just saturated my imagination and created me to explore more of this touring around the city.

So, I stayed over at a pub that night again but not the same one as before, having a coke, and off to bed what more can I ask for? But what I liked more about it was the fact it was on the main street of Waterford where I was stuck looking out at all the lights imagining how everything was built into place like I always did growing up. The next morning I was tired and was thinking I might head home as I didn't feel well and felt seizure auras coming for a few hours. I was only across from the bus station, but I said forget about it; I may as well at least reach as far as the ferry just to say I've gone that far, so off I went that morning and had just missed the ferry to Wales. Then the feeling of seizures began to worsen. So, I went for a walk on the beach saying to myself that it doesn't matter where I go ill still get them. As long as I have this condition, I'm only going to punish myself more, and on the other side then, I've family and friends worried sick about me due to having it probably wondering where I am all the time.

You know, I just needed a different atmosphere to be in and not be in the same dark place where I only end up dwelling on everything. Everyone around me keeps reminding me that they're talking about my problems worrying about me hoping I'll be fine, which made me feel like a problem more than a person.

Anyway, I began to walk back the N25 road towards Cork and said I'll head home and hit London some other time, so off I went back home. Once I got back, I said to myself, Maybe I should have waited for the next ferry. But, I was happy to be back in Cork for now.

A few months went by. I used to miss the family life and talking that went on at home. It was just a small touch of loneliness, but I knew deep down I was better off out of home due to the level of worry going on when I lived there. So London was on the menu again.

One Saturday morning, I packed my bag and went to the holiday agent in cork and got a ticket from Cork to Heathrow airport in London. Then, I rang a few friends from different parts of London who I knew only a short while and told them I'll be there later if they like to meet up.

So, off I went to Cork airport, rang my mum telling her I'll be in London for the weekend, but I told her not to worry and I'm meeting with friends there and it's only the weekend I'm going for, and she replied (I wouldn't be surprised if you were in Rome meeting the pope at this stage). So I laughed and got off the phone then when I was arriving in London for the first time and didn't know what to expect, the size of the place shocked me compared to all the other places I had been in so far. So, once I arrived there, I got the tube train through the London underground from Heathrow to Seven Sisters and found a small hostel nearby and stayed there for the night.

Then, I met up with a few friends in Covent Garden, and we hit the cinema nearby where hallways through the film I felt another seizure come and it did. I was at this stage wrecked tired from a week's work and after coming to Lon-don, and having another seizure, but people around me didn't notice it because it was only a mild one and in the back of the cinema, so I fell asleep and woke up towards the end of the film.

They said to me when the lights went back on after the film, "Seems you weren't very fond of that film," and I went along saying, "Yes, the start was okay but lost interest after a while." and laughed.

So, I had my way of getting around things when I could if I felt it was better too. I was okay then once I hit the fresh air again, and we all went to Leinster

Square and took it easy for a while. I asked one of them who was from London were the most dangerous place in London that you wouldn't go near on your own.

He mentioned some street close to Tottenham and I became interested in going there on my own been as daring as I was to see what all the fuss was about where people can't walk certain streets on their own.

So, we then decided to separate for the night and meet again in the square sometime tomorrow. Off I went to this place that was supposedly dangerous the next morning as I had no problem going anywhere on my own like that.

So, I was walking down that street, and yes, I did sense a bit of tension, but I wasn't scared and went into a pub there that was full of dark people. As I walked in, they all stared at me as if they were saying to me, "You are not meant to come in here."

So, I walked up to the bar and kindly asked for a Red Bull and sat down, and they all got back talking to each other and minded their own business. There was also a pool table in there, and I put up money to play next. This big guy was playing, and I was hoping I wouldn't be playing him because it looked like he took this sport real seriously. I said, "Jeez, I'll just have to let him win, or I'll be destroyed," so he beat the other guy anyway.

I said to myself, Well, I'm up! I went up.

We shook hands and said whoever wins gets £10, so letting him win was out the door at this stage. We played anyway, and it was a good game, but I just managed to beat him and was surprised I was all wrong because he put down the cue, handed me a £10, said good match, shook my hand and walked out where I was expecting a dramatic reaction.

What I learned there was not to judge someone by how they look just like someone shouldn't be sympathized with what they have. The reason you get looks from all these places is that you believe these people are trouble when not all of them are, so they're going to start causing trouble if you don't stop giving them a bad name judging them. I went across the road then to an Irish bar where I played more pool, and there was a guy in there from Belfast who I found interesting. We started talking about London, and I said someone told me this street is dangerous. He said it can be like last week the window of the pub was smashed in and three people came flying out the window.

I laughed and said to him, "I thought those kinds of days were long gone," and he said to me, "He's a black belt in karate and also a boxer."

And said, "That's the only reason he can stay and go out there."

Did I say to myself, Go away your joking with me? but I didn't mean it like that. I just found it amusing how someone would have to go to the bother of defending themselves to be around one street in London, but I understood his point of view at the same time as he lived there quite a while and I didn't.

We were playing pool, and I asked him why he came to London and would he ever go back to Ireland. He said he loved Ireland, but living in Belfast was not a life to be in then, which I didn't understand either since I was never there but only saw Belfast on TV.

I said, "Is it as bad as they show on TV with what happens up there?"

He said, "If you can live in Belfast, you can go anywhere."

That was the reason he began to box when he was younger because he said you must look out for yourself living in a place like that. Anything can happen at any given stage.

I thought seriously for once and said to him, "Didn't think I'd ever say this but I don't have an attraction to go there because of how you described living there and the fact someone like you who goes out in a dangerous part of London isn't living there."

So, I never went there since I had no reason to go there but was tempted to a few times and it felt like no mistake meeting him to make me more streetwise. Later on that evening, we exchanged numbers and said our goodbyes, and off I went back to the hostel for a while. Later that night, I met up with the group of friends back in the square, headed out clubbing

with them, and at this stage, I was still not drinking
So the night went on, and everyone had a good night.
Then, the next day, I flew home to Cork and fell
asleep on the plane as I was wrecked and had a mild
seizure again on the plane going home but was not
noticed, but it was a good weekend with a lot of
interesting people I had met and a lot learned. Then
another morning when I used to do a lot of cycling
like the times I was washing cars and windows and
had built up to over 100 regular customers, it was a
sunny summers day at 6:00 a.m.

I said to myself, I think I'll cycle to Killarney, which
was about an hour's drive from cork and a very well-
known tourist area in Ireland like the song (buried in
Killarney). I went and got on the bike and cycled
away. I was very fit at this time as I used to be able to
cycle a kilometer per minute on a straight road.

As I reached past Ballincollig two hours later, I had a
seizure on the bike and fell into the bush. I was
wrecked tired after having one and again like I said
earlier began to put myself down. However, I
recovered and said well I had one now, so I should be
okay for another few days. I cycled on and reached
Macroom and took an hour's break there and then
went straight on to Killarney and was there by the
night.

I felt I achieved something again, and it felt good, so I
said I may as well book myself into a hostel and stay

two nights after that. Off I went and did that and went out that night.

I met a lot of foreigners and told them what I did that day, and they were surprised and said not many people my age would even go to the bother of walking a mile never mind doing that, and well done for doing it. I said thanks and said thanks but I'm not cycling back and could sleep for a week after it now. They laughed and said I can see that.

A few hours later, I went back to the hostel and must have slept twelve hours straight till I got up. I hit the road and was debating whether I'd cycle further to Dingle. I didn't, but I was full of energy, and the more I had, the more I expected from myself. But, this time I went to the bus station, threw my bike at the bottom of the bus, and headed back to Cork. Down, I had this happiness in me, which was describing me as happy to have done something again that I would be labeled as not supposed to do. I got back to Cork, got off the bus, took a deep breath, and said, "Yep, now I understand a bit of what freedom feels like, and it's really good."

I used to thank God for helping me get home safe and sound and still be in one piece and used to always wonder if someone was looking over me watching my back. I think what I'm trying to say here is I began to understand why the parents were always worried and began to slowly mature in myself especially the fact I wasn't living at home anymore. The tour-ing around kind of cooled down for a few years as I was more getting used to the fact of planning a new life after the operation if it still goes ahead too.

I was doing a lot of thinking. My oldest friend Nigel used to always say you're thinking too much because I'd be no use in his company and go all quiet and start thinking sometimes. The imagination takes over once the boredom starts and relates to thinking and wondering.

Like I was saying, so I cooled down for a few years because different things began to happen and different people began to come into my life. I was a bit of a home bird since I was going up and down to Dublin for nearly two years that filled in the travel side for me, but at least I knew Dublin by now too.

One time I said to Derry□who is described in a later chapter□how I met him that we should both go to London and Make an adventure out of it at the same time only making conversation with him. The next thing, he replied saying he would be interested in coming too, which I thought would be even better for him due to the fact on his way back from there many years ago was when his illness began from the tumor he had.

This time at least he can look forward to good things happening when he returns, so that was planned. I went off up to Cork, got the tickets and two days later we went on the bus from Cork to London. I just loved been on the move because it relaxes the imagination and feeds the imagination to develop more creativity and Derry was also more artistic than me.

That completes me when I'm in that atmosphere because it also puts the mind at rest and the imagination to work. Off we went that Saturday heading for London by bus from cork and reached Rosslare ferry that night and headed off to the top of the ship looking out, feeling the sense of freedom and allowing the breeze to create a special atmosphere like it was the right thing to do at a time like this and go enjoy it. We went down, had a few drinks.

Surprisingly, the ferry was quiet enough for a Saturday night and once we hit Fish guard in wales, we were checked for ID. Then we all went back on the bus and headed straight for London. It was a long journey, to be honest, sixteen hours in full as it was my first time by bus to London.

We pulled in at Victoria station that morning about eight a.m. and I was shattered. We looked for a hostel immediately to get a bit of sleep. We couldn't find any, so we walked around to the taxis. They didn't want to drive because they were so near, so they just gave us directions.

I knew from there and said to myself This is going to be an issue, so we followed their directions, which led to nowhere, and I said, "The hell with this; we're in the middle of London, so let's just grab a cheap hotel."

We were a bit tired of each other after the long journey. I was worse than him because I didn't sleep a wink since Saturday morning. So, we found a place, which cost fifty pounds each, that was perfect because we were there in the morning and didn't have to leave till the next morning.

So, twenty-four hours for fifty pounds each only comes to over two pounds an hour, which sounds good to me especially a hotel that included breakfast.

Off we went and both got to sleep and went out a few hours later and had an early night in the hotel bar later. The next day we went to find a hostel, and he came up with a clever idea of taking the hostel yellow page out, so we started ringing them. I found one by Earls Court, which wasn't far from where we were going to be getting the bus back. So off we went, found it quite easy, and signed in there for fifteen pounds each, which we also showed up early at so was well-worth fifteen pounds. Then we split as I went off with my CVs and went around London to Strafford where the Olympic stadium was been built and gave them a CV and threw in a few more to different parts of London. I was glad to get that out of the way.

We went out that night and had a way better night because we got to know a bit of the city and were not getting lost anymore or overtired, so everything was at ease. The next day, which was a Monday, and the last day, things were still kind of busy in the city; and we found out it was a bank holiday there, which was good to hear because it was also a nice warm day.

Everyone was happy to be off. We went and took some photos of the statues and bridges and the London Eye then went around in the tube to different busy areas, and took some more photos, and went on a bus tour around the city. I just couldn't get my head around how big this city was and how in god's name I didn't see it the last time I was there. I suppose it depends on whose company you're in too.

As night came, I was highly fascinated with the lights at night there which were massive compared to other places I stayed and could just stand there for hours watching them flash if I was alone but don't think Derry would have been too interested in it as I wouldn't expect him to be even though he was also an artistic person. So that was the London tour.

The next evening after seen more of the city we went to the bus station, got our boarding tickets in Victoria station, and waited for the bus that night. We went off back home. I just wanted to sleep the whole way back. But for my friend, Derry going back was a really special part for him and indeed more of a gamble to take as he said the last time he was on this bus going back from London was when his seizures began after having a seizure in the toilet of the ferry another 13 years followed.

I thought he might be anxious going back, but he just had a smile on his face not caring about it, so it was grand. When we hit the ferry, we walked up to the bar. I saw the toilets and said, "Well, do ya need to go?" He said, "No, but I'll go in any way to wash my hands," and I said, "Yes, put a final closure to how all that chapter started, and I bet you'll have some strange news come to you once you get home since this for you is total closure to how everything started," and he agreed.

Surprisingly, he did get news when he went home that he was offered a temp. job for a few months, which was a new kick start to a new part of his life. As I got back to dun lock, my hometown, I was glad to be home; but I sensed that I needed to go away again soon. Cause I've done the work thing and college thing, so I promised myself once I came home to concentrate on going away soon rather than work since everything was quiet in Ireland then and I've worked hard for so long even during having the condition.

I may as well do a bit of traveling and find work abroad at the same time in another part of the world if possible. I needed to specify whom I was and what I wanted in life now, so I needed to see new places that were not possible.

All those things would have been just blank places to me before whether I went or not. Now, as I'm running wild into everything looking for anything creative and imaginary, I was happy about going. I began to surf the web once I got home and my friend

Cyril who I lived with told me about a train that goes all around Europe that his niece went on.

I searched that up and it was cheap because first I already had a bus tour planned since I picked up leaflets in London to where I can go from there, which was more or less anywhere in Europe, but I was questioning myself wondering if I'd be able to go for it by bus, which I probably would but not all in one go.

Inter-railing looked like it was going to be my next step on touring after Cyril telling me it was meant to be great and he would come if he had the time too.

The next destination I wanted to go to was Prague in the Czech Republic after doing a course in college with a girl from there who I saw was very artistic and good at what she does too. I for some reason think it's the architecture that captured me there too, and also I wanted to visit Slovakia with its landscape and buildings.

I began to also look at ship routes from Cork to France, and the train seemed to be the more advanced and suitable way of going. I was on my way to plan another European trip and to go on my own as I had friends who probably would come. But, they wouldn't be too interested in going to the places I wanted to see once we got there and many were too busy with the dates I had set. I said I'll go alone. Music also played a massive part in this journey, feeding the imaginative feelings creating the atmosphere as if I was creating a story or movie in my head. Every song I heard when I was on the move, I could create into a story or develop into a movie in parts depending on the tunes of the song and where I was passing when I heard it.

In the cities, less can be created because everything is there; and in villages and small towns, creativity was big, and the space and lack of negativity were there. The nicer the landscape, the calmer the imagination would be.

A week after coming back from London, I got itchy feet again and drove to Cork and got another return ticket to Lon-don but was going on my own this time, so I got the ticket, met up with Derry in Cork, and told him I was off again. He said I was mad to go that soon. I said I know, but I need to get a few things done and maybe also finish giving my CVs out to certain destinations I planned to go to last time to see if I should go live there. Off I went a few days later on another night trip to London and was more equipped and knew what to expect, so when I hit the ferry, I got a cabin and did some writing, took it easy, and had a shower to wake myself up. Back on the bus then and I got to sleep from Cardiff to London.

I was fine when I got to Victoria and got the tube as far as Earls Court, which is only ten minutes away, and hit the hostel I went to last time with Derry, which was booked out, but they were a great help. They showed me a hostel across the road, which was only two minutes' walk away. I went overbooked in around nine a.m., but booking time wasn't till twelve.

I saw another group from Munster there but said nothing even though I knew one of their faces. So I just left my bag there, Then as I remembered Nigel's eighties party was on the following Saturday and everyone had to dress up, so I hit Covent Garden since it also had a market there. I got my friend Maria something who I was planning to visit the next day up the country, as her birthday was that day I arrived.

The T-shirt I got for the party had all colors and a tribute design on it. I bought that for Nigel's birthday party and went for a drink. Then, I went back to Covent Garden, sat down to watch the musicians, and ended up leaving my top there only realizing it twenty mines after I left when I was on the tube.

I didn't forget Maria's present, so I was fine as I believe what you lose something it will return in some other way. Off I went back to the hostel, took it easy for a while, and hit the public house across the road, which was good, and I enjoyed my own company for once and had a few drinks there.

Nigel texted me asking how I was getting on. I had no credit to text him back, so I went to the Internet cafe across the road after the pub and told him what I was getting up to and that I expect a damn good night Saturday after buying stuff for it twice after losing the first one.

Maria texted asking if I had any place to stay that night and gave me directions where to go, which was Peterborough. She told me they can pick me up from there so I rang her and left her a message. I said I was grand for that night as I booked a hostel earlier and will head up to her in the morning. I went back to the hostel for a bit of sleep; out for the count I was at this stage from seen a fast life there and around eight a.m. I got up, hit the road, went back to Earls Court to Victoria on the tube, and asked there how to get to Peterborough up the country from London. He said you go directly there from King's Cross, so I got the tube to King's Cross and booked a return ticket to Peterborough.

I was off again and rang her around eleven a.m. From there telling her I was there. She rang back after she told her mum and said she'll pick me up in about an hour, so I waited there. Her mum picked me up and I was off to meet Maria whom I knew nearly nine years but never saw yet.

I got there, which was a country place just like where I'm from myself, and we just talked and talked from there for hours. Her family welcomed me in, and I just felt grand as I wasn't sure what to expect in the first place, but everything seemed to click into place when I got there. I caught up with Maria on everything we used to share, and she showed me pictures I sent her before, which I couldn't stand looking at because I wasn't a happy person in them. Then we said we will go into town and take a look around, so off we went and did some shopping and hit the bar after that.

We wondered why the hell we never got to meet for nearly nine years after I made some attempts in the past but never seemed to make it. "Now so many things changed in my life, and I finally meet you I said." And she said the same, so we had a few drinks that day and just talked all night about our beliefs and wants in life and got half-drunk in between all that as this was later after I had got better which is written later in the book. Finally, we called it a night about seven a.m. or should I say morning, and were up again at ten. I for some reason was grand, and we went off to Peterborough City where I was getting the train back later that day.

I said my goodbyes after meeting a good loyal friend Maria for the first time and everything that happened man-aged to go smoothly and fit into place.

I said my goodbyes and said, "I'll see you again soon." I got the train back to King's Cross in London, got the tube to Victoria, walked to the bus station there, and booked my return ticket back to Cork. Before the age of 32, the 20 countries I have seen were England, Scotland, Wales, France, Czech Republic, Bosnia, Croatia, Italy, Netherlands, Germany, Turkey, Kazakhstan, Australia, New Zealand, China, South Korea, Spain, Yugoslavia, Switzerland, And Luxembourg.

So, as I said before do not leave the system impossible and neglect yourself from it cause that's how it works where you are, and believe in yourself that you can take control of your path and goals and things might start to happen for the better. If the system does not work for the better of you go and beat it by creating your one because everyone is a corporation so many should take back their own rights when they are not met for the right reasons.

Paganism and divination

The word occult means hidden knowledge and if you ask me, I think anything that's hidden is worth checking out to see why it's hidden in the first place — just like elite people are always hidden away from society when they are the people creating the massive systems people are living and working in.

Here, I'll explain how I began to learn through the inner-self system that can reach any limits of spirituality from its previous experiences of learning and experimenting. Psychics who I went to out of curiosity for future events or happiness have in some way led me to believe certain events that only fitted my character.

I only went out of curiosity not a predicted future as that would have become a very boring life to have it all predicted and if it was predicted, I would have reversed it due to it been predicted because you can only make the decisions in life, I believe. So, I learned very quickly about the difference between the con artist psychics who tell by looking at your character for clues and asking specific questions to manipulate you to explain something they can simply answer, which eventually shocks you. Some psychics shocked me telling me exact stuff I've previously lived through and guiding me down a road I could take.

Since the age of thirteen, I used to have many flashbacks that began in foreign countries like at events of celebrations, and sometimes these events would tell me that something is soon going to happen; something like a wedding or some sort of celebration that would usually involve friends or family or even people I had only seen. It would also link to certain stages of their lives where they were in jeopardy from their previous way of living or in trouble with mortgages and so on. It was like intuition but stronger. It felt so positive that I was very right about whatever I thought. I would just be very much alert if something was wrong, and there was no manipulating me, trying to convince me that everything was fine and level. These senses were way too strong to just be a motion, and this sense began to grow as I got older and had a come-and-go appearance in whatever stage of life I was living.

Here's a perfect example where I once sensed that my parents had serious financial problems as the house possessed problems or bankruptcy; not that I knew exactly what it was but was on a level to know that something big was going on, pretending everything was fine.

It wasn't as if they were arguing or were any less materialistic or that no food was on the table, because everything seemed to be fine and normal at home.

But, I had this huge weight of worry on my back that something wasn't quite right like a mother does and can't help worry about her kids. I was around sixteen at this time. I used to tell my friend Nigel what I was feeling and he didn't know what to say at first, but the more I thought about it, the more I wanted to find out what can be done to fix the situation I was feeling.

Spiritually, I just began to grow from here, which linked me deeper into thinking of solutions to everything and search deeper within myself. I and Nigel used to talk about our futures and dreams and began to wonder what our futures would be like.

Everyone does, in general, all that kind of dreaming, and he had certain things like tarot cards, which was mainly for the sake of redrawing the pictures printed on them, and told me these could present my future, and when I asked how, he said he didn't know yet, so we let it be.

Shortly after feeling this weight for about a month, we left the place we lived in, which, as I previously mentioned, was a house above a pub in Saleen, and moved two miles closer to Cork and got a bungalow and restarted life there. After that happened, the weight was off my shoulders and I wondered how I was getting these incredible strong senses.

I was drawn into all this spirituality. I began to think I finally was getting answers to things. I was linking them to other limits that I was always looking for. Nigel told me about a white witch who lived in Cork some twenty miles away and that she predicted things and could tell the future, not tell anything bad.

I was humming and wondering for a while and said I wasn't sure about things like that. He said it didn't sound great, but I knew someone who had grown up with her and she told her things that had all happened.

I was told not much before this by our local priest to stay well away from these sorts of people. But, I was also becoming more lost in myself and didn't think I'd ever escape from epilepsy and depression, thinking I would soon die, so I went to her at the age of eighteen as I was adamant about getting answers and thought what can I lose if I was just curious. She brought me in and sat me down, asking if I was over eighteen, which I was, and read my palm. Then, she said there is something about surgery to cure something you have at present.

I questioned her, acting stupid, and said, "What do you mean?"

She said, "No, you'll be fine when you reach twenty-two, but till then struggles will come and go that will only make you a lot stronger."

That just made me lose total interest, so I wasn't happy with her at that time and believed it was all a load of false crap. I went away from the psychic interest at that time for a while until I started thinking more and more deeper, wondering more and more, and struggling more. I looked deeper into where my life was going since I started to panic more about the future, taking on more responsibilities when I felt I had enough of my own.

I'd never give myself peace of mind on where I can lead for a destined future. I saw this ad on TV about Irish psychics live. I rang them one day to see if it was a hoax; night upon night they told me all the things I wanted to hear that sounded so helping and great but can easily become so addictive as sex talk can for sex addicts.

I was getting addicted to hearing such great things from my mental health starting to deteriorate from tension due to the pressure I was putting upon myself. I was in a fantasy dream and for that split moment, everything felt fine with all the great stories they were telling me and my consciousness was at ease until I just got totally and utterly hooked after about a week. I felt I was getting answers that I needed, rather than wanted, out of desperation that I was going to be cured. Of course I never even thought of how much credit I was wasting because I was too out of touch, hearing things I wanted to hear and being manipulated into their business!

Money didn't even come into my consciousness. I even used to go to payphones and ring them, spending all the change I had just to hear those simple gestures that, you'll shortly be out of this mess you're in. This enabled me to finally imagine something positive, just to hear that good things are finally going to happen. This over-the-phone reading was a total scam, just like sex lines, or some women who demand everything and give less and vice versa with men.

It shouldn't have been licensed at all and should be completely banned as it ruins people's consciousness and becomes like drugs, making them search for their next fix, especially if you have any addictive personality problem or ADHD of any sort. You would be hooked on it in no time due to the way your consciousness differentiates fiction from the faction. So these senses I still had were still not leaving. Every time I heard the phone ring, I could picture who it was more than the name who it was. Most of the time, I was right but not all the time. Someone I haven't thought about in a long time would automatically just pop into my memory, and all of a sudden, I'd bump into him/her the next day or even later that day or get a call from him/her. I also had funny feelings around my stomach when I sensed older people who were close to me as if I could tell rather than presume that they didn't have a lot of time left to live here. Then I began to have dreams, which would appear to flashback in front of me like déjà-vu the next day.

I just learned not to take it too seriously at one stage and just don't let it brainwash me, ignore it and it might go away. I tried to structure my thoughts so they made sense, but every time I was looking for answers, this was the only way I thought I found them as it created a sense of direction and clear consciousness.

So, I went to a psychic in Cork when I was twenty, as one afternoon I was up there and saw a sign just beside Burger King for a psychic who was once on the Late Late Show. I was surprised that such people were allowed on TV, and he also did the first five minutes free. I rang the number and booked an appointment and at this stage, just hoped everything in life would be strong, hoping I could just take my own life back.

I wanted to know about my health issue, of course, and work and told him nothing, acting completely stupid like I was new to such an experience, so off he went, dealing the cards and all that. In terms of your health, he said in a toned-down voice, "Right, it says here, there will be an operation coming up."

I didn't have a clue what he meant, and I replied, "What? Operation!"

He said not to panic though because it will bring great happiness and will be a complete success whatever it is for. I wondered, the light switched on — he was talking about the epilepsy been cured.

In terms of money, he said I'll be going from job to job until I find what I'm good at and that I will be very good at it and stick to it and have incredible creativity that I should start to use more. He then said, "There are loads of talents in the bottom of you that are crying to come out," and, "Soon, you will develop them one by one," and, "Structure will create progress in your life and lead to a career even though you already have abilities to succeed financially."

Finally, he went into friends and relationships and said I'm going to soon meet someone who has very similar characteristics and needs and who will be in the same position as me. He said that we are both going to help each other out and become very good friends. He will also be very creative.

I walked out of there assuming all this was to happen at once since I was very impatient and didn't know what to believe even though he shocked me with how he knew many things that he was never told anything about. I didn't look like I had anything wrong with me either or acted as I did. It all happened when times were right for it to happen, bit by bit. He was spot on, and I only copped onto it when the events happened.

Another night, when I was out in my local pub☐The Rock☐there was a famous UK psychic above it that everyone was queueing up for.

I went to him probably at the age of twenty-one since everyone else was going. He took the front of my hands and started talking about my present feelings, which were rough, and said, "Things are finally about to take a turn for you. But, you won't emerge to see it till you begin to lift your spirit. An awful lot will happen over the next few years, so be prepared for many new events," and that I "will live to tell a story."

Then, he went on to the heart and said I have a solid heart and will never get any sickness or injuries and will succeed in life emotionally. I asked him to tell me more about the past as I wanted to believe him.

He looked at me and said he doesn't have to prove himself to anyone. I laughed and said, "Fair enough." Then he said things are not very good right now but, "All you have been through will be returned to you in time…"

When all that he said was over, I went to another psychic a few years later, whom a friend I met in Dublin from Cork told me about. This was the same person that a previous medium in Cork told me about a few years — Derry, who was also creative. I was twenty-four, and she also shocked me with many things she said. She first got me to deal the cards, and she said to throw down the first seven, and I did. She asked, "What do you want to know about?" which was the usual question.

She said someone was always worried about me, which I presume was my mum with all the things I was up to, but she had calmed down quite a lot recently, which was probably because I was finally better than before.

She said I was very bright in terms of designing, which is probably my main aspect and should be working for myself too but give it time as I also get bored easily. She also asked whether I had ever thought of doing signwriting, which I had only

206

applied for a few weeks before this, so I laughed and said yes.

Then, she said, "Well, you're going to go ahead and do that and go ahead and do something similar afterward that won't interest you in the end," which I did do. It was graphic design.

She said after that I will begin to do something that I'll be good at and that is painting and decorating and many other things, which also did happen soon after. Finally, she said that I will be writing something in the papers and for radios and make business cards that will be funny too. She said I will do well and surprise myself. She mentioned that she could picture me in a van and that things will work out. She also said in terms of relationships, I'll meet someone out of the blue whom I already knew but haven't seen in quite a while, and things will lead from there. But, what she said was, she might be abroad.

She also said that someone in the family will be going through a tough time soon but will get there at the end, which also happened. Lastly, she said whatever happens in life from here on will never be as tough as before. She also said that I have very strong abilities too and whatever the case, next year will be a great new year, which it was.

I started a relationship on New Year's Day, started college three days later, flew through the course, and moved in with my partner at the time.

I can't say that wasn't true. She finally said, on the last note, to give me a little time and space to redevelop things and not to rush into anything as everything will work out in the end.

Soon after, I began to have very strong dreams; as I was in control of everything I ever wanted through this year, I had similar ones every night.

Once I was in a plane flying it through a storm and land-ed it perfectly fine; and next, I was driving a blue lorry going full speed ahead on the main road; and in another one I had, I was steering a hot-air balloon with my eyes focussed on its landing.

Everything began to run smoothly, so after hearing all this good news, I came to a point where I thought that I should no longer go to psychics and now continue to lead my own direction and use some of what they told me as directions if any of what they said occurred later.

I decided it was now time to seriously stop because if I didn't, it would just become an addiction, and later I would lose full control of myself if I continued to just go to them because my goal in life was always to just be an artist and become enlightened if it was ever possible.

I knew deep down God did exist and he was much bigger than whatever can be predicted and much purer, so I should leave all worries to him and not allow myself to get caught into a predictive state.

Therefore, I reversed all the people who did come into my life that were predicted.

I didn't allow myself to be with them since they were predicted to be with me by these psychics. Also, I reversed work and went to places that I just decided to go to on the spur of the moment and not places they told me I should visit or would suit me better. So, all the good things that I was told about were happening, I reversed and this way, I took my destiny back and started from knowing nothing again.

This time, I felt much more in power than in the dreams I had and it felt incredibly liberating to finally be in full control of my destiny, not knowing what could be ahead.

This is dangerous and just as manipulative as Predictive Programing is and should not be played with like it's just a bit of fun as it programs someone to open up to dark forces who live in deception deceiving others when they think they are helping others. They are not they are destroying others' lives. It is an entry to witchcraft nothing more which dangerous world leaders would only love to use as the dominant world religion.

Finding the cause

At the age of nineteen, the breakthrough had finally come a few weeks after I came back from Medjugorje. This is a holy place in Bosnia in south-eastern Europe, where our Virgin Mary was said to have appeared sometime before, which I believe also had something to do with finding the problem.

How I went on that holiday was not out of luck but felt like it was meant to happen, because I used to visit the local priest just a mile down the road some Saturdays to wash his win-dows and clean his car for him.

One Friday night, I decided to ring him and ask him if he needed anything done on the weekend, and he replied that he was okay with everything for now but thanks all the same. He said that he was actually in the middle of a meeting at the moment so he didn't have much time to talk.

Then, he stopped for a moment and said, "Actually, can I ring you back in a moment about something else if that's okay ?" and I said, "Ya, no problem," so he put down the phone and phoned me back an hour later. He asked if I was ever in a place called Medjugorje. I said, "No," as I didn't have a clue where it was and had never heard of the place.

I asked what kind of place was it.

He said there was a group of them going there shortly in a few weeks, and the meeting he was having earlier was about who they were going to bring as they had a free ticket which included flight and accommodation. It's over in Bosnia, next to Croatia, but they would be flying to Split in Croatia and get a coach the rest of the journey to the hotel.

He asked if I wanted to go, and once I heard that there was traveling involved in it, I said, "Ya, no problem, and thanks," so he said to call over to his place tomorrow for more details, and he would tell me all about it and what to bring.

I got off the phone and said to my mother, "I just got invited to go to a place called Medjugorje by the priest," and she asked if was I going to go.

I replied, "Ya, why not?"

She said, "You know, that place is a bit like Lourdes in France. My parents sent me there when I was around fourteen with a group. I felt a little awkward there, but I liked the place itself in general but in terms of how holy it was, and the belief people had hoping and praying scared me a little at that time."

How many people depended on their belief felt a little like mind control to me back then. I looked at that place as a holiday because I wasn't yet giving up because of what I had and wasn't putting all my faith in one place where I saw no solid proof of miracles in the first place except a few people on crutches who could walk again after going there. I've seen worse people in psychiatric centers looking for second chances too so I was not fully convinced having seen a few crutches in a place that probably made a fortune from tourism.

I thought to myself, This place is amazing in terms of structure and it must cost a fortune to maintain it but must also make a complete fortune with how many come here! as I was still young enough too and had not fully entered the materialistic world of illusion and peer pressure completely. But, I did see Lourdes as a developed place for people with issues to indulge their experiences, create a new consciousness for themselves while they're there and gain a new experience. But don't be brainwashed about the place; go there believing in yourself. I said to my mum, "I'll go for the trip to Croatia to see the place more than go there to be healed."

A few weeks later, I went with a group of people, some of whom were sick and some going for other reasons, but we were all from the same town and outskirts. We flew from Cork to Split Airport and got the coach from there to Bosnia, where I saw rows of houses bombed and blasted to pieces and wondered, "How do people manage here?"

Seeing all this misery and foggy depression just opened my eyes to a new world of wonder. By around three a.m., we were at our destination, and this certainly was the destination that did something for me. I loved the place. The weather was great and people were more down to earth, and the way of living was just getting by and not materialism.

I remember one particular day when I was in church and was in a queue of people to get healed by a priest who was meant to have healing powers. A friend of mine from home, Jane — who had also come — was in front of me and when she went up, she fell backward from whatever he did to her.

I said to myself, This can't be true, so I was next, and he did the same to me. I didn't fall backward but did feel much better after he touched my forehead. The only thing I can remember that everyone got after it was that they couldn't stop laughing as there must have to be something in the air. It was endless. I also knew Ashley — whom I was sharing the room with as he was a brother of a friend Jamie back home and also had the same condition as me — but we didn't talk about it much, as it took enough of our time away by having it.

Soon after that, I had a seizure down in the lounge. People from the group were a great help and helped me back on my feet after I woke up and they brought me back to my room. A few hours later, one of them who was a massage therapist gave me one of her treatments, which was a great help.

I was back to normal for now and went on a walk around the town in the middle of the night just to see all the lights on and the peace, which I always liked to see, and no one was about. Then the next morning, I rang my mum at around nine, forgetting they were two hours behind, so she was not happy.

I told her that it was a great place to go and the people were nice here too. And a few days after that, it was time to go home, and I had another seizure and was tired of getting them again, so I was looking forward to going home anyway. I said thanks to the priest for his help and support, and that hopefully, it may have done something for me and the rest of the group too.

Then a few weeks after that, I had an appointment in Cork Medical Centre again. They decided to take me off a drug called Rivitrile since I was on it for so many years at this stage and was becoming very dizzy the past few months, so he said to go home and, "We'll call you soon when we have a bed ready for you and will change your medication again."

I said in a tired tone, "No problem."

I waited and waited. Weeks went by. Months went by, and finally, they called when I was at work in Cork with my dad. They said to be up there that Friday night, so we finished up the job and went home early that day, packed my bags, and went to Cork Medical Centre to change my medications. This was usually the main reason I was staying in there most times.

This time, I acted out for some reason and I was pleading with the doctor who was a new member of Dr. O' Donohue's team. I wanted him to realize how bad my mood swings were from the medications I was on and hoping that whichever ones they were about to put me on this time won't be as bad.

I was explaining how often I was getting side effects and that my consciousness was going crazy and just to watch me and the new member of the team said to me, "I don't think there's anything wrong with you. I think you have it all in your head at the way your acting and you're only looking for attention," and that I should get psychiatric help.

He had the very same attitude as the vice-principal did when I told him the situation in school when I ended up leaving school. I just took a deep breath from being misunderstood once again. Then a few hours later, he came back over and said to me that Dr. O' Donohue had decided to book me in for an M.R.I. scan (Magnetic Resonance Imaging) in the university hospital the next day. But if I asked him, it probably will be no help at all.

So I looked at him and said to myself, I'd love to put you in my shoes. You're playing with someone's future here, you don't have a clue what you're saying, and you expect me to listen to someone like you. There I was with no idea to look at and a screwed up consciousness full of negative thoughts and traumas and he was a medical doctor telling me I've no hope, saying an M.R.I. scan wasn't going to find me anything. I was only imagining everything! I was fired up to the top with rage hearing this from a so-called medical doctor as if he had been in the situation himself. I could have punched him that day with rage.

The next day, I had the M.R.I scan up in the medical center where you lie down in a tunnel and they slide your whole body into it and you stay still holding a panic button while they turn on the scan. All it does is shake and was about five minutes long.

After that was done, I returned to my room in the other hospital. A few hours later my doctor came over to me and said they have found scar tissue by your left temporal lobe on the left side of your brain, which is good news because it may be a possibility for surgery and has a high percentage of being cured.

I didn't have a clue what to say after been told by the other member that it was all in my mind and that I was the problem and then this was told by the team leader.

I didn't know what scar tissue was but was glad that they found something for me to look towards at last, and if anything, it just didn't seem to register to me right away. I asked if I could look at the scan, and the doctor said, "It's just an x-ray and a scar tissue is more or less a lump of tissue in your brain that's no use but is probably triggering off the seizures since

216

medications have never seemed to work for you and made you worse."

I said fair enough and was happy that I got an answer and began to wonder what the next step was going to be and started to get a little excited too at the same time.

The doctor then said to me he's going to transfer all of my medical files to Dublin Medical Centre and from now on and I will be going up there from here on and will let me know who my new doctor will be soon and that I won't need to go to Cork Medical Centre for check-ups anymore. Now, it's all about seeing if I can get surgery to remove the scar tissue, which may take a few years of tests and could be a long road. For most people, it changed their lives around completely, and what harm is in it to give it a go and see if they can do anything for me.

I was delighted that I had some bit of structure forecasted on this condition I've had for so long now. I began to make new plans already as I was getting excited about maybe having a new life at some stage. Then I saw the doctor coming towards me who said it would not find anything, and the shame on his face for him to be wrong said it all. He didn't even congratulate me or apologize for him been completely wrong. He had just walked by with his head down when it was usually up. Just because doctors are intelligent and supposed to be there to help us doesn't mean I'll never find a narrow-minded person like him with a serious attitude problem but if he wants to be a doctor.

All I say today is I hope he learned a very hard lesson that day because if he was my team leader at that time I wouldn't have had the M.R.I scan and could still be looking for answers and would probably be on a suicide mission by now or else in a bar trying to drink myself to death.

I rang my mum and told her they found something, and she was only over the moon. They came up and sat beside me with a big smile and my mum said it took twenty years to get this far! Twenty years of torment! I just nodded, not wanting to look at it like that because I was happy that they found something. On the way out of the medical center, I asked my dad what's scar tissue because I wanted to know more details. He kind of got annoyed as if I should know and bluntly told me but was also very annoyed that it took this long too.

I mean I was happy for once in my life and it just sounded like they were putting me down when I'm there trying to hold on to a bit of hope and get an overview on what my chances are of looking at a future.

However, I think my dad was mad at the doctors for it to take so long to find something positive and was tired that we now had to start another chapter realizing my childhood was damaged creating problem after problem due to this scar that was in my brain.

I sensed that he thought he failed and should have known or brought me for an M. R. I. years ago. When it could all be done and dusted by now.

Well, that's the impression I sensed anyway, but I hope he didn't feel like that because he was still there all those years for me trying to brighten me up and make me see sense, but I was too stubborn and lost to see any of that.

I just wanted to move to the next step as soon as I could, so I got back from Cork Medical Centre and was put on a vitamin folic acid. After I got out of Cork Medical Centre a few days later after a week's work, I was back on my travels.

I went up the country alone the following weekend because I needed to clear my head and understand what was happening right now in my life.

I went back up to Cork and headed to Sligo by bus and stayed up there for a few nights. It was summertime and I was up there before working. I was walking the beaches up there at four a.m. in the morning, which reminded me of Medjugorje but on a different route, and was wondering what was going to happen if I was cured and how would I deal with it or all the things I will be able to do?

What would I do with my life when it won't be as challenging anymore. But, I stayed on the negative side too cause I still had a long way to go and it's way too early to keep my hopes up. I might still be told I'm not a success for surgery as I had loads of tests and appointments before that can be said. I went to a beach I was once in due to work, that was called Strand hill where there was also an airport and just took in the sense of freedom as I may have to get used to it and I had sat there all night long listening to the waves crash off the rocks and watched the planes take off and land and worry-ing didn't even exist.

The next morning I walked back to the bed and breakfast where I was staying and Nigel rang me asking if I'm calling down to him. So I said I'm actually in Sligo and he replied, "What the hell are you doing up there?"

I told him I needed a few days alone and will be back Tuesday, and he said, "No worries, give me a ring when you're back!"

Then, I was up at the taxi base later that day and asked if there was any other beach like Strand hill around? So, a taxi brought me a few miles away to a place called Rosses Point just outside Sligo, and it was a lovely sunny day, and this place just took all my thoughts away immediately. I felt I was floating in a calm atmosphere with nothing to worry for or about. It was even better than Strand hill, and I did the same kind of thing there and could picture myself going back there again in the future. It was a place of healing for me. I pick up on atmospheres very quickly and know whether I should get out of there or not like how intuition works, and this place was just the perfectly calm atmosphere for the time I was in then.

I stayed another night because I wasn't just able to say goodbye just yet since it felt right. As soon as I got back to the bed and breakfast, I wondered why twenty years of my life, which was my whole childhood, was lived the way I lived it and then find something in my brain that's been causing it all along. I was angry with how long it took to finally get an answer, and annoyed that it couldn't be done there and then, and believe me, I'd almost another three years of it left, but over-whelmed that they finally found what was wrong with me and I wasn't a basket case after all. So put the three of those feelings into one combination, and that's how I felt then.

But that was only for a while as I was alone and had nothing more to look back on. I wasn't sure whether it was way too early to think too positively. I finally sensed freedom the weekend at the beaches up there. I was not used to good things happening and ran back to my past every time I felt out of place or that I shouldn't be feeling too positive. Soon after this, my consciousness began to wonder too much about how much of a difference it would make if it was possible to be cured and maybe a new beginning will start that I might be too overwhelmed to handle.

Then, after that, I went back home to Cork and was waiting for my first visit to Dublin since I felt I was ready to finally say goodbye to epilepsy. A few years later I had found out Derry was also once up here and we took a trip up there one weekend and that weekend he met a guy from the same part of cork city he was from that had just moved up there.

Dublin medical transformation

This was a chapter where everything I had learned up till now was forced into perception and put into proportion to finally do something about it and everything had fallen apart completely that felt like a nightmare but it happened for life to become easier.

A new and final chapter of my previous life began shortly after the M.R.I scan, which is how they found the scar tissue in the left temporal lobe of my brain at Cork Medical Centre.

It was the final and most stressful road to recovery that I couldn't even imagine I was going to face. I knew that everything was probably going to have to fall apart before I get better for the next chapter to begin. All my previous characteristics and interests were all grouped into this chapter alone that made total sense as to why I was the person I was and had to be that person I was.

It was a sudden death road to another life, so here it goes. I got the first appointment to go to Dublin Medical Centre early in 2001 when I was twenty. I and my mum went up for the first time in a time where I was leading into depression from emotional stress. I had a lack of knowledge about what I was up for through this entirely new chapter with new doctors, new tests, a new hospital, and so on.

An understanding of everything was poor, with the side effects increasing, making me almost unaware of what stress even meant anymore since I was in that state or whatever other state of mind I was in I was unaware due to experiencing it at the time I could not ever manage to explain it.

All my experiences, characteristics and tactics had been built up inside me from years of feeling misled in a failed health system so in a way you could say the health system had a disorder too and not just its patients. As I reached adulthood, I was looking back and tried to see if there was anything positive that ever came out of this. The more I looked back, I was like an experiment trying medications, and my mind was going backward rather than forward with measures of hormones colliding with actions of rare dysfunctional illusions on who I even was or what I was.

I said to myself, "I am not going to let the team of medical professionals experiment on me in Dublin like I have allowed them to medicate me like crazy in cork the last twenty years.

I know well it was the medications as if they had created some sort of bipolar effect throughout the years when I was forced to take cocktails of them rather than just one amount. I was extremely angry towards how our health system was un-regulated here and the failure of communication in all aspects between medical staff and patients who were not private with no private insurance. They were treated poorly as compared to those who had private health insurance. At this time I couldn't talk for myself anymore as I had silenced myself from depression. The only thing I did not need help anymore with was been fed or going to the toilet but other than that I was very old-looking like I was on the way out simply from depression. I was also tired of trying to succeed in everything and get ahead of everything rather than just survive in the here and now. I couldn't stop seeking to get better and get ahead of the game along with seeking knowing there has got to be more to life than this all at once. My mum had done all the talking in Dublin Medical Centre this first time we went up to where I just sat there staring into space and wondering what was next.

But it was way out of my league to function straight and understand anyone anymore. The depression was becoming worse and I had lost a lot of weight too and stopped eating properly.

So in other people's eyes, I had a bit of an attitude problem towards new people who were trying to help me and another one with myself which was not a very smart move to make at all.

Or, in other words, the more drama I created about whatever was going on in my life, the more some people attracted themselves into my life. It felt horrible that these kinds of experiences can make other people feel much better about themselves or more secure which states maybe it is them that need to be medicated with something.

Then again countries treat each other the very same way by debt and if they can`t afford their debt there are always possibilities of war and blowing each other to pieces.

I guess that's a lot worse and makes an awful lot less sense too when you think about it so knowing that people were attracted to my experiences had me feeling like an object more than a person. I didn't get the last laugh for quite a long time yet and hearing people worry and talk about me behind my back only made me feel twenty times worse as it made me think, "Have all these years I already went through shown how much I can cope with?"

Rather than having people worry, I would have preferred people to just tell me not to give up now after this long, cause worry just creates more drama and another downturn and never creates any solution to any situation.

I gradually lost all confidence in myself due to hearing that over and over for years. It had just drained me out, and also just ignored the people who were talking out of gossip rather than those who were concerned. People's lack of understanding was quite exhausting for them also, as they were trying to understand and communicate to the guild in whatever way they were able.

But, that's a level of knowledge that can never be shared, as the levels of frustration to the person experiencing it and the person educating themselves about it are never equal, like those fighting a war and those watching or reading about it are not.

However, the sense of failure that came with the depression from my lower self-getting the better of me became emotionally draining, and guilt on my department that I withheld for years due to the failure in all the systems I entered. I kept giving myself a hard time fighting against it until I found the solutions to whatever I was looking for.

So, the first time in Dublin, Professor Jack ward was the first neurosurgeon I met there that day who was also the team leader and I remember waiting out in the waiting room beforehand feeling a seizure coming. I told my mum I felt like I was going to get a seizure, and the aura kept coming, which always happened before the seizure. My mum then replied, "Maybe it would be good if you had one in front of the neuro-surgeon so he can acknowledge it more in detail."

I replied, "True, doubt it will happen then though. In the end, the auras just kept on coming, which was also normal, but I never had any seizure. Finally, after waiting for about two hours, my name was called by Jack Ward.

We went in, and he sat us down introducing himself as Professor Jack Ward who will be the leading consultant from here on, and asked, "What's the situation and how have I been since the MRI scan in cork?"

Then my mum responded to him saying, "The seizures are still as common and he is becoming more depressed," and she took out the medications I was on and showed him.

He just looked at her and replied, "I don't need to know anything about medications," shaking his head, "I just want to know how Eddie feels about surgery more than anything to finally put a stop to all the years he has had epilepsy?"

He also stated that his doing surgery is nothing new and that it's not something anyone should ever worry about as he has been doing it for a very long time and does not get stressed from it or any bit unbalanced.

He added that he would like to question me if that's okay since I was the one who has the problem. I woke up when I heard him say that as someone might listen to me for a change because no doctor ever had that attitude towards me, interested in what I had to say for myself before. A doctor who would just listen was one I was always looking for rather than medicating me again or judging my behavior to label me with something else.

I even looked around the room when he said it just to be sure he meant me because I was depressed and was a little bit out of touch.

He was quite a funny character, who started going on about Cork at first, and the football, and how much he missed Cork as he is originally from there himself. I was sort of smiling and laughing and saying to myself be this the guy who will be operating on my brain if I'm the right candidate?

He came across as just some random guy you would meet in a public house and have fun with so my nerves had be-gun to completely ease from meeting someone in his position with such a different attitude than the rest I have come across.

I was expecting some stuck-up highly intelligent arrogant man telling me a load of stuff that sounded like complete double Dutch, which was what I was used to. But, then he started talking more seriously and asked me about how I felt about surgery if it can be done and what kind of upbringing did I experience growing up with it?

To be honest, I didn't fully remember at this stage because my mind had taken over from traumatic stress so much due to the emotional stress.

It was strained to remember anything long-term and was more or less in isolation so memory was gone long-term including all the trips I had done around the country and people I knew or met along the way. They were swept clear out of my mind at this point and any good things that happened or that I enjoyed were completely forgotten too as these are the effects depression creates. It dubs down your memory sort of like some people who get rich can forget where they might have come from or how they got rich in the first place and what life was like before they got rich, etc.

He then started going on about how long I could be coming up to Dublin for tests, which is bizarre in one way because I used to travel up frequently before for no reason anyway. But, then again it is the capital and the biggest city after cork.

Maybe, I was meant to get used to this route anyway. He said that the longest I should be waiting will be one and a half years max due to the waiting list there is at the moment with all the tests that have to take place.

After those are all complete, I will be transferred onto a waiting list for surgery if it's a success to go ahead, but could not tell me an exact time limit that I would be on that for, and if it was successful recovery time would usually depend on how to fit you are but it's usually only a few weeks to a month before you are completely back on your feet.

Usually, it is also advised you should take a year out of work or whatever you are doing to more or less get your life back on track as it can be a complete change for some and very overwhelming for others depending on how long they had the condition or how immune they were to have it.

Everything began to sound positive for once, but in the back of my mind, I didn't want to get too excited because this was only the start of it and I had loads of tests to get over and done with before I could be told if I was suitable for the surgery.

I couldn't imagine or even get excited about being cured at this point, as I couldn't see that far ahead anyway due to the severe depression. It erased anything positive to be accepted into my consciousness and created a cloud of isolation, guilt, and shame.

I always knew from that day that once the surgery is done and I believed it would be at some point as I thought. Otherwise, I would have seen myself as being completely cursed so I believed my time of having this would finally be over and it will be gone for good if it can be done so that was my final straw to hold on to.

It also explains how the mind works in many different strategies. It was like a gut feeling telling me you must hit rock bottom and lose everything before you get what you need rather than what you want.

Some can be told that it would be too dangerous to operate on them due to where the problem is located in the brain after all the tests. That to me would be way too much to take in even though it's just the reality side of it and does happen I don't think I could have taken it very well if that happened to me.

I went back to Cork that day not knowing what to expect when I was to come up next time to Dublin. So my behavior got more settled and calmer ever since I knew some sort of new system was in place now.

A few months later I was called up again and was happy that something different somewhere different was happening.

I was a little bit confused and did not fully understand what scar tissue was or how it had got there in the first place, or what they meant by the problem been situated on the left temporal lobe. Due to falling into depression for a long time and becoming manic with concentration at an all-time low, I had a very poor mentality to function clearly.

If anything, all that was on my consciousness at this point was ending the atmosphere my mind was in. I know for a fact it was the Neurontin that had changed my ways of thinking and created much more damage and despair.

I had begun cutting myself when I was on it also before becoming suicidal on it next. I more than likely had to begin researching everything bit by bit to understand what was going on and what`s going to happen to me the way things are going. In some way or another, try and reactivate my mind from thinking to re-learning and re-programming. No matter what the risk of the operation was, I had made up my mind a long time beforehand that I was going for it.

I've tried for so long to live a normal life with it and just did not fully fit in somewhere, and that just was not happening so whatever they could do to cure me of the position I had been in throughout childhood my life was worth the risk.

The next appointment to Dublin Medical was to meet the neurologist Dr. Norman O' Connell - Professor Wards researcher - who deals with all the research, medications, tests, and so on.

This time my dad had driven up. We were waiting in the waiting room for about an hour and were called in. We both came in and sat down as usual and he asked how I was feeling since the last time I was here and I said grandly as I could just predict what was next.

I was sick of the same questions over and over so had a bit of an attitude problem. He started concentrating on how often I was getting seizures, which had become more frequent. He asked me whether I throw my right arm or left arm to the side while I'm having a seizure.

I said to him I don't know what I do, to be honest and looked to my left towards my father hoping he would answer the question. He said that my left arm starts to spasm and jerk up to the top then my head would repeat to jerk to the left too. Then, he asked what type of seizures I was getting and my dad said most of the time they were absences but can sometimes get grand malls too. From what the father was telling him, he was just nodding his head as if he had a good idea of what he meant and what medications I should have been on, and what ones to try from here on.

All these trips to Dublin with one of my parents were beginning to annoy me the fact I had got to a state where I could no longer fully look after myself and it made me hate myself more and more the more someone was helping me in such a state. The next time I told my mother I will go up on my own in the future since I have been coming to Dublin anyway since I'm eighteen. There is no need for anyone of you to go to the length of trouble to go all the way to Dublin and back whenever an appointment comes up. They knew I was my person and was up there numerous times before so they said fine and my mum had a sister up there in Malahide who was my godmother☐Annmarie☐ where I could stay if I wanted to and that was that solved.

A few months later, another appointment had come up and I went up on my own and felt a lot better in myself and was not at all tensed and bothered because I felt more stable going up alone. I was more used to doing things alone anyway and was also the one doing the talking from here on knowing that it was between me and the doctors whatever it was about now.

I was up for an appointment with Dr. O Connell again and he asked how many seizures have I been getting since he put me on Keppra and took me off the psychotic Neurontin that drive me mad.

I told him at the start I had a few grand mal seizures but then I was okay for a few weeks, which is surprising since just over a month was the most I ever had without one as far as I can remember.

After that, they continued as normal again regularly but there were no side effects like before, which was the main thing. He then put up the dose of Keppra from 2000mg per day to 3000mg per day. He made sure I was still going off the Neurontin at the same time, which had completely stopped by the time I was on the 3000mg of Keppra along with Lamictal daily. Lamictal was the longest drug I was on at this time and was on 400mg per day of that per day and also 300mg of Epanutin per day and these were more or less the last daily drugs that I could more or less try. I was on everything else that was on the market anyway for someone in my condition.

But, at least I had an open option that might someday cure me and always tried to keep on the positive side knowing that too. I left after a few minutes. He said I'll have another appointment in a few more months for my memory that was called a Wada test which was named after Canadian neurologist Juhn Atsushi Wada□or also known as an intracarotid sodium amobarbital procedure - I.S.A.P.

After I went home that time All of a sudden, I didn't hear from them for months upon months nearly up to over a year for this test, and began to feel anxious and wonder if they have forgotten about me or what was going on.

But, about six months later I had an appointment again in Dublin but with a psychiatrist this time - Dr. Sandra Throughton - for my depression and memory loss to keep me up to balance.

So, off I went up to Dublin again and met her for the first time and got the same usual questions on how my behavior is and how I was feeling. She made the atmosphere feel a bit calmer as if she was a friend and not just a psychiatrist so I felt a lot calmer than I normally did with previous ones I had gone to before.

She went into detail on how I felt about myself, as my confidence towards anything had been going downhill rapidly from emotional stress to depression. She asked if I was worried that surgery might not work to see how much I was holding on to the negative side rather than the positive and all those kinds of tactics.

Like I said I was not bothered about any of the risks but was very tired of playing the waiting game same as someone who can be in desperate need to be enlightened and go through anything to just achieve it. I was getting more stressed as time went on. Boredom began to develop due to all the things I've already done and played my part in the process.

She asked me if I would rather see a psychiatrist in Cork than have to come to Dublin for those appointments along with the other doctors too?

She made things one bit easier, and I replied, "Yes that would be a good idea." She said she would make an appointment for me in cork with a local psychologist to go and see her regularly and that was the first and last time I had seen Dr. Sandra Throughton. I went back to Cork that day and was glad I could see one of the team now in Cork rather than Dub-lin.

About two months later, I went to Cork and met psychiatrist O' Sullivan. She was more interested in herself being right about everything rather than getting to the point of finding the issues that were creating me to become lost and depressed.

She was doing her job right in her strategy and got some points right about me having behavior problems and been quite stubborn and some wrong with what she has done with medicating me been the psychiatrist she was who came across someone desperate to be a doctor.

She wanted to know so much all at once and made me feel very uncomfortable when she asked me to tell her everything and realistically was not listening to the way I was feeling and immediately felt I had to be medicated due to my depressed state and attitude.

She began to work with my G.P. Dr. O' Brien who was my local doctor through childhood. She stated to him that she thought I was in urgent need of being medicated with anti-depressants. It just reminded me of Dublin Psychiatric Centre all over again, not knowing what sort of way they would make me feel or whether I would be put back into such a place been on them.

I was highly stressed by now and far lost from anyone could even imagine. My manic depression had taken its toll. I was fading away like a leaf and looked like a complete zombie. My mental health was literally about to snap. She decided with my local G.P. to put me on the anti-depressant right away called Cipramil, which I was not sure if was a positive thing. I was already on many medications for epilepsy along with vitamins due to lack of calcium that was due to all the other medications I had been on over time.

The local psychiatrist in Cork and my local G.P. Dr. O' Brien more or less agreed to try a few that should be safe enough for me to take and put me on one that was called (Cipramil), which at the time did give me a very big boost for a while.

I had just moved out of home at the time again too with a few friends into town as I needed time away from family with so much happening in my life all at once. The Boose Cipramil created also came with a price of downfall and after about two months on it, I was so sick of all the medications I was on that I felt like a walking chemist.

I said to myself, "Screw this I'm better than this," as the seizures had also got worse. I believed the fact I don't have to be treated for depression; I can sort that problem out myself without been medicated for that too. From that day on, I stopped taking them immediately. For the next few days, I felt a lot better than I believed I did the right thing.

I knew it was simply a relapse and that I would have some very serious side effects on the way soon to allow it to detox out of my system. Around a week after I stopped taking them, I began to feel like I just wanted to slice my throat as slowly and as painful as possible and gently and free flow my journey to hell there and then if that is where I belong due to the life I have been set to live through. So much confusion and disappointment of coming back to this planet of deep error got in the way.

I could not think straight about doing anything stupid living in a backward world even though I could not fully think clear. See, you must bear in mind all these thoughts are in your mind at once. A few days do not lead up to it, but all at once. It could be all the frustration of all the pain that happened in a few months to a few years. That's when the person will literally snap as the mind can only process so much negativity before it shuts off. So much positivity before it becomes overwhelming at once Someone can more or less end up brain-dead or relapse where the mind will have to rewire itself, which can be like the same process of someone healing from been heartbroken. That's one reason you see a lot more people hooked on drugs or sex, or worse scenario dead from suicide, due to not be able to handle the relapse that can create an evolution within the person.

A mind is a serious machine that can lead you down any path at all and I believe your mind is the atmosphere of your body. You can either live in illusion by it or live your destiny to succeed in your own life on your terms rather than been programmed. A few days later knowing this was a relapse, I was fine and all that feeling of wanting to commit suicide in some way was gone but I still didn't go back on the anti-depressants. I knew willpower could help me a lot more if I was to allow it. Not to be led to rely on them that I would be less depressed if I continued to take them daily.

The next appointment with the psychiatrist in Cork was a few weeks later and I told her I gave the Cipramil up because I didn't want to rely on them for any comfort of being healed.

However, I was still stressed and deeply depressed again but was not as bad as the first time I went in to see her. She urged me to never do something like that again without telling her first and wanted me to go on a stronger anti-depressant than before. This time the fact I came off the other one, and the new one was called Effexor and I said, "No, forget about it I'm done with being treated like a walking chemist and I have had enough."

She replied it will be the last one and to just try it for a month at least and not repeat the same thing?

I finally came around and said ok to more or less put a stop to her nagging conversation. As the appointment was over I went home not wanting to take any more drugs but did promise to try this as the final one. It was like a sleeping tablet to me after about a week, cause every time I sat down I fell asleep and slept during lunch at work. My dad said, "You better move home if you're like this all the time."

I just had no energy to eat and went straight to bed every time I got home. I had to be woken the next morning for work again as I was even beginning to miss my medications every night without the energy to eat properly too. I was someone who had gone hibernating. My mum got very annoyed seeing me in this state after coming back from work every day and said that "This has got to come to a stop! Because he has no living being on these anti-depressants. He's sleeping every minute of the day he gets."

This didn't matter because I didn't feel like I'd have much of a life anyway. I was enjoying the little time out I had.

The Effexor was no help to me and I went back to the psychologist and told her that these are just putting me to sleep and reminds me of Cork Psychiatric Centre that I was in before for the same reason and seeing most people in there like zombies. She wanted to send me to a more up-to-date psychiatric center in Cork to put up the dose of Effexor because I just wanted to cut myself from being so stressed along with the new side effects from it. I had been asleep most of the time.

I was still getting seizures every few days and trying to keep a normal job and living out of home all at the same time. A week after the appointment that day I was in Cork Psychiatric Centre voluntarily, and they began to put up the dose of Effexor doubling what I had started.

The effects got worse I couldn't feel a thing or eat a thing or even to that matter talk to anyone or had zero sex drive both from depression and the effects of this drug which was meant to be a treatment for depression yet causing me to be much worse?

I had weighed twelve stone when I went in that time and within a week I lost a stone from the effects. I felt like a para-lysed individual that week.

I was still getting the basic questions every day like how my feeling and I felt like smashing all their heads in at once from their stupid basic questions and wanted to so bad say what does it look like to you? What are you going to do other than treat me with more medication to stabilize my moods?

She recommended I stay in there the week and see what happens. The days went on and I was only getting worse. I began to wonder why do I bother listening to her as I couldn't even go to the toilet properly at this stage. I also couldn't feel anything happening in my genital area. My worry became a wonder there. I decided I don't want to be here anymore as it has done me no good and signed myself out the next day with everyone in the hospital and at home telling myself it might be best to stay in and get help. I said to myself, "What help?"

I was sick and tired of listening to others and signed myself out. I also stopped taking that medication to the point I felt a higher power of courage that came down my spine for a few seconds due to finally being able to stand up for myself bit by bit. I was getting away from all these people who called themselves medical professionals that had caused me more issues than anything.

After many years of listening to others and going along with what they were saying in detail, I had enough of it and went home feeling a little better about myself. That was the end of taking any anti-depressants for good, which took some time to detox but the only place for them with me was the bin.

I was done with them at this stage and began the process of coming off them which took a few weeks. When I think about it now, it just shows the power of the mind; that it can do absolutely anything when you leave it and it's the most difficult part of us to control yet the most simple to manipulate. That was now all out of the way, and I had quit going to the psychiatrist in Cork from there on and felt much better for being allowed to make the decision myself.

My parents had advised me to go back to her and continued as it might be part of the process of being allowed to receive surgery in the end in Dublin. But I replied, "No, I have had enough of her now and do not need to go there again or I will be outraged at her for the conditions she has already made me face." My parents, at the same time, we're also going through a phase where they were not sure how to communicate with me anymore. They knew at the same time that they could not force me into what they thought was better for me anymore and that I had learned to make my own decisions now.

I had more or less learned to drift myself slowly away from anyone who worried about me because I did not want others worrying as there was way too much going on all at once to explain over and over to everyone who was concerned. Now, I had the anti-depressants and psychiatrist in Cork out of the picture. I was soon on my next appointment up to Dublin and this time, I was getting the first set of memory tests done, like quizzes and numbers and matching comparisons. All these were to make sure that where the dam-age was activating in the brain was only in that spot and that my memory did not affect it.

They could tell by my answers whether I was on the right path and if I would lead onto the next test. And the quizzes were things like putting puzzles together and making words with certain letters and asked a few maths questions too. I passed them all.

Off I went back to Cork that day, wondering what was next on the agenda and a few months later was called up to see the neurologist Dr. O' Connell again, so I got the bus up from Cork and a taxi to Malahide the night before and stayed at my aunt's place.

The next morning, she drove me to Dublin Medical Center and I went in to see the neurologist who said he was now going to offer me the Wada test soon since I have passed all the current tests. This test is where essentially, a barbiturate (which is usually sodium amobarbital) is introduced into one of the internal carotid arteries via a cannula or intra-arterial catheter from the femoral artery.

The drug is injected into one hemisphere at a time. The effect is to shut down any language and/or memory function in that hemisphere to evaluate the other hemisphere (half of the brain). Then, the patient has engaged in a series of language and memory-related tests again. The memory is evaluated by showing a series of items or pictures to the patient so that within a few minutes, as soon as the effect of the medication is dissipated, the ability to recall can be tested.

I went back home on the train to Cork that evening and waited for that next appointment, waiting and waiting for months upon months, getting sick and feeling like moving abroad to the U.K. at one stage, just to get away for a while and clear my head.

So my mind was relapsing with anxiety and frustration from playing the waiting game again. But then, over six months later, I was given an appointment to see Norman o Connell again and get the Wada-test complete.

The second he injected the chemicals into my thigh on my right leg, my consciousness completely froze and I was not able to speak.

I knew what he was showing me but couldn't tell him because my speech had frozen more or less the same way it does when someone just regains consciousness after a seizure where your speech is broken till you fully come around.

I was also laughing at the same time from the effects of the chemical, so about thirty seconds went by and my speech was beginning to come back. They asked me the same questions again on what they had just shown me, which were simple things like pictures and numbers and shapes. I got them all right so Norman more or less started to nod and say, "Yes he seems to be fine and suitable for surgery by the signs of it."

He looked around the room to the rest of the team to see their reaction and they agreed the Wada test was passed with flying colors, and I was fit to go through the surgery.

I think the decision on going ahead with the brain surgery was made thereafter a clear result.

After I finished, he said to me that my very final test coming up in Dublin was going to be an E.E.G.☐Electroencephalography. "This is where we are going to keep you in for around two weeks at the most and will rec-ord you twenty-four hours a day. We will monitor the levels at which your brain is operating and wait for you to get a seizure or two. So, we can see what happens to your brain when you go into one."

He told me that it's a more equipped CT scan that gets more information on what's going on and they attach all these wires to my head and inject needles into my jaw to read the level of nerves coming up towards the brain.

He then said to me that there's quite a big waiting list for this test and there are only two beds in Dublin that do it in all the republic of Ireland so he couldn't give me a specific date for when I would be called up for it.

I went back to my aunt's place after the Wada test and told her the story and stayed there for the night as my leg was only half functioning due to the injection.

The next day I went into Dublin city from Malahide and got the train back to Cork. I was drained from trying to take all this and not fully understanding the process of what's happening next. I was just getting more tired every time I was coming up and was more or less ready for any risks at this stage. At least the news was starting to get more positive than it ever was before, even though my patience was running out.

Then I got back to Cork and went home and told my mum a brief story on what went on and just sat there hoping the E.E.G. will come soon as I was very much ready for it now in my consciousness.

Again I waited for months upon months, more or less another seven to eight months should I say. I was so bothered as I knew this would happen again with the structure of our health system here. I felt like we're being abused because of what's wrong with us or you could nearly call the sick the forgotten ones but at least I had been pre-warned this time. After seven months, I was at my friend's place a few miles away. My phone began to ring and I looked over at Marie and said to her, "It's the hospital. I know it is."

She said, "Answer it."

It was them and they said there's a place for you in Dublin Medical Centre for the E.E.G scan this coming Tuesday so I said, "Thanks." I told Marie the story and she said that's great news.

Then I went back home and told my mum and said I must go up Tuesday in a calmer way so she wouldn't get too excited about it. A few days passed and I was on the train to Dublin again and my mother came up with me again since I was going to be staying there for a while. We got off the train at Houston station and got a taxi to Dublin Medical Centre. We went straight to reception to check-in and were sent up to the room on the first floor and I walked in and it was a small room with only two beds and a toilet with a small room next door for a full-time nurse to make sure everything was okay. The nurse welcomed me and said a guy from Galway had just left from the test today. She asked where I am from. I said Cork and she said I should have known with the accent and said your roommates are from Cork too and I looked over and said hi and that was when I met Derry who was also artistic too and in there for the same reason.

So I got settled and my mum stayed in Malahide that night with her sister and I got all the wires put on to my head and had blood tests and got needles put into my jaws and was put on a drip.

My mother left soon after I had been wired up so I said goodbye to her and she went to her sisters. After that, a friend of another one of my aunts came in with her daughter Annmarie who I didn't know at all.

They introduced who they were and said she had this done a few years ago as she also went through all this and she told me she was my aunt's friend. She said she would pop in to say hello since she heard I was here so I got to know her and her daughter Annmarie. They gave me their number and said to stay in touch and soon left so I kept in touch with Annmarie from there as she knew the whole process herself after going through it herself.

As the night had drawn I got to know Derry that night and asked him how long he had epilepsy and how bad does he have it? He was a bit slow in replying due to his previous seizures the day before and said he has a tumor and said he has it twelve years and I asked how come they only found it now?

He said he went to England to re-abolish himself because he was being nursed. He felt he needs to wake up and try something himself to help himself and when he was in England he was brought in for an M.R.I scan in Manchester they found a tumor by his left temporal lobe. It has been growing and causing the seizures all those years and sent him home to get it removed as they didn't have his files there so couldn`t do much more for him.

He said he went home after back to the cork with his sister Sa-rah who had been nursing him and living with him as his carer all those years.

She got on to his doctor in Cork who brought him for an (M.R.I scan) there in the same place I had it but had not found anything so they decided to transfer all his files to Dublin Medical Hospital after hearing that and told him to go there for now.

About an hour later after he finished telling me his story I was talking to him again and got no response. I looked over and he was getting a seizure where his whole body began to look like waves upon waves coming in on a beach.

He was about to fall off the bed onto the floor so I caught his body and his head and put him down on the floor. I pressed the emergency button as the nurse had just left five minutes earlier. She came flying in with a few more.

I told them he just had a seizure and they shut the curtains and began asking him questions like who's the president of Ireland and all that. I said to myself, He is not going to be able to talk after a seizure your consciousness has to come back together along with your memory before you can speak properly again!

He was looking at them side to side mumbling not being able to talk properly like I can't either after one.

I asked him as he came around about an hour later if the nurses do that all the time and he said yes. I then asked him how long has he been coming to Dublin Medical and he said a year and I said I've been coming three years. Then he asked what part of Cork am I from and I said dun lock and he knew it since he knew it wasn`t far from where he was from. So we were getting to know each other. We ended up having a lot of interests in common. It didn't even click that I was told a few years before about later meeting someone similar who will have a lot in common with and will help each other out by a medium. But, it was good to finally meet someone with the same challenge from the same place knowing that I wasn't the only one suffering this from the same place.

So, a few days went by and I still had not got any seizures and Derry had another one and was told he will be moved to another room the next day since he had enough now and they have monitored enough information from him and he was suitable for surgery to remove his tumor.

I began to get anxious and said to myself, "when you want them they don't happen like the first time I went in to see neurosurgeon professor ward. But when you do they won't and was worrying about maybe being sent home after two weeks if I don't get one cause of the list there must be for this place the fact there are only two beds in the whole country for it. I hoped to God I will have one since it's the final test.

So the nurse tried to get me to cycle the exercise bike that was there for that purpose to cause a seizure from exhaustion. I knew there and then that it wouldn't work for me because I had done a lot of cycling in my teens and it never caused me to have a seizure so I said no I'm not doing it as I already saw Derry on it and he doesn't think it made him have one either.

I said why not take me slowly off my dose now like you said is the idea if someone does not have seizures in the particular time limit you normally expect. They decided to take me down on one type the next day, which was Epanutin that I had been on the longest and took every night. The same day Derry was left out and moved a few doors down to another room.

That night a close friend from Cork Kenneth and his fian-cé Claire who I knew for years at this stage and now lived and worked in Dublin came to visit me. I said I was still waiting to get a seizure and as soon as I do will be let go and that should be the end of it. As soon as they were leaving Kenneth said to me "never thought I'd say this to you Eddie but could you hurry up and get a seizure? I was laughing and said that shouldn't be a problem! That night they put my dose of Epinutin down once again and I had numerous seizures all in that one night

I even remember waking up in the middle of one and saw Dr. O' Connell and a few nurses there trying to stabilize me and then they began asking me questions when I was coming around, which I couldn't answer as my consciousness and memory were not fully functioning yet.

The next day after I came around I was relieved that I had the seizures out of the way and Derry was going home that day and we exchanged numbers and promised to keep in touch so he went home to Cork that morning.

I was told by staff I had three seizures that night and can also go home the following day. So I got on to my mum and told her that I can go home tomorrow but am thinking of heading to Skerries for a few days since it was also the weekend and I met a new friend Annmarie who was after getting this done a few years ago and was welcomed to spend some time there. So I signed out after seen doctor o Connell the next day and he said all you have to do now is simply wait for the call to have surgery all your tests are complete and you're suitable for surgery.

I shook his hand and thanked him and said no problem and was so much calmer due to meeting two other people who had the surgery and was also going to have it. I went into Dublin city and got the train to Skerries town.

I texted Annmarie asking where to go and she explained it.

I went along the beach and cleared my head. It reminded me of the time I spent in Sligo a few years back when times were a lot darker than they were now. Skerries was a nice place too just on the opposite side of the country. I just sat there for a few hours taking the fresh air in and seeing the beauty of nature that costs nothing again. I stayed at Annmarie that weekend and we became friends.

Then, after getting back to cork a few days later Time went on and on again. I didn't hear from anyone about anything and thought I have forgotten about it again so I was getting annoyed and decided to start ringing the medical centre my-self after about eight months and got no answers.

I managed to get in touch with someone who was able to give me Professor Wards' office address. I wrote to him saying that I think I've had this for long enough. I went into detail about it, and what they said to me, in the start, about waiting a year and a half, at the most, where it was over double that time at this stage. I also said, I know and understand that your profession is very stressful and demanding. But, I also know that however long it took you to become who you do not make up the time I have had what I have. I can't control it.

 I wanted some sort of response to what I posted and when I could be seen.

Then, just over a week later, a letter had come in the mail from them, which just shows that you've got to fight your corner here to get an answer. The letter more or less said, Thanks for the letter and you will be seen as soon as possible, as talks about your surgery are being currently scheduled so expect a phone call in the next few weeks.

So I said to myself, No problem at least they got back to me. I didn't contact them again. Then, a few more months went on. One Sunday, I was with Cyril, an old friend from school down in West Cork, and my phone rang. It was a private number.

But, I knew right away that was the call I was waiting for and I said to Cyril, "It's the hospital." He said, "Answer it, answer it."

It was and they said, "Come up by tonight. The operation can be done tomorrow morning."

So, Cyril rushed to the closest town, which was Kinsale, to get a quick bite to eat.

I threw my spare change into a plot machine because I wasn't hungry and I won over a hundred euros after throwing in two euros. It was a lucky day for me!

I rang my mum telling her they called me and I must go up tonight. It was all a rush at home too, to get my stuff packed, so by the time Cyril had dropped me at my home, my stuff was ready. My Mum dropped me straight up to the train station. Just before I left, my dad said, "Come back better, Ed, and best of luck."

I took a deep breath, shook his hand, went to the train station, and said, "Good luck" to my mum there. I went straight to Dublin Medical Centre.

I got to the medical center and told the receptionist the story that I was meant to stay here tonight and be operated on tomorrow. She said that they were out of beds and were not told anything about me coming up tonight. She said that she did see that I was on a list to get the surgery done tomorrow. She asked me if I had any relatives or someone I know where I could stay tonight and come back in the morning.

I shook my head and said, "Yes, but I was called earlier telling me directly to come up tonight."

She said I must have misunderstood because there weren't any beds available. But, I was seen by another doctor, who just took a blood sample, and told me the surgery was on the list for tomorrow but there were no spare beds for that night.

I rang my mum and told her the situation.

She talked to her sister about it, rang me back, and told me to get a taxi to my aunt in Malahide who is also my godmother. She said that she will drop me at the medical center on her way to work in the morning.

I went out of the medical center and stayed in Malahide for the night. I explained the situation to them too and was dropped there the next morning. I was also wished the best of luck by my aunt that morning.

So, I went back up and was told to wait here for a few minutes. The doctor who saw me for a few minutes the night before called me in, asked me a few basic questions, told me to get undressed, and gave me a throw-over.

I was waiting in a waiting room full of people and he said to me, "I'm just going to go find your M.R.I scan." This was the scan I got in Cork over three years earlier. I said to myself, Oh. Don't tell me this is going to be a problem, as I felt that it could be, and it was.

He came back and said, "Well, I have some good news and I have some bad news. The good news is we found you a room for tonight."

I knew what the bad news was, but asked anyway.

I was right.

They couldn't find the M.R.I scan results of the scan I had in Cork, but wheeled me down to the theatre anyway, while they were searching for it. They said that if they didn't find it, they'll book me an M.R.I scan there in Dublin Medical Centre as soon as possible. But, the machine was being fixed at the moment.

I was a little distressed and tired from all the rushing and tearing around and then I hear that. Of course, I wasn't surprised either as I was used to nothing being perfect, which can't always be expected either. Now, I was down in the theatre, not knowing what to expect, and I just couldn't wait. I saw everyone else being wheeled in taking into surgery for whatever they were getting done.

I asked the nurse, "Do people often wait this long, as I have been waiting?"

This was over an hour later and she said no and tried to calm me down and asked if I wanted something to drink.

I said, "No, I'm fine. Thanks." Then a few minutes later, a load of doctors came over to me and surrounded the bed.

It was the whole team that I had met throughout my time in Dublin. The neurosurgeon Professor Ward came over with his team. He said, "We're sorry but we can't find the M.R.I scan from Cork but I will operate on you this Thursday as you can get an M.R.I scan here before then."

I replied to him, "Fair enough but you are going to operate on me though, aren't you?"

He said, "Yes, not to worry we just need to see the MRI scan before we can start."

So I said, "Fine."

My consciousness had been put at ease after knowing that I wasn't going to be rejected or sent back to Cork to wait for another appointment. I rang my mum. Her phone was engaged, so I rang my father from the theatre room, and he was shocked to hear from me, expecting me to be in surgery.

I told him, "They can't find the MRI scan. I must go for another one here and can be operated on on Thursday. I have got a room."

So, he got on to my mum and she rang the medical center in Cork where I got the MRI first and she got back to me, saying that Cork Medical Centre said Dublin Medical had it.

259

I got off the phone and told the doctor that Cork Medical said it was here, just as he was walking into the room. He said, "Yes, we found it now. It was put into the wrong colored files and your name was spelled wrong. But, now that we have found it you don't have to go for another M. R. I. scan here. We will get on with getting you better once and for all."

It just shows how a small little mistake can become a mess

I rang back my mum and told her that and she said okay and was relieved everything was back on track for surgery. I was going to roll myself on Thursday and was getting geared up for it by talking to everyone I saw, telling them how excited I was, without even knowing who they were.

They said they would be scared to death if they were in my shoes having brain surgery.

And I said, "Well, whatever happens, will happen but I've got nothing to lose anyway and everything to gain so why not go ahead with it."

I got to know them over the next few days and Kenneth came in Wednesday night with his wife-to-be, Claire, and wished me the best of luck and I said cheers to her for that.

My godmother came in too and said, "Best of luck."

I said, "Thanks a million, and thanks for everything."

Then, the big day came on Thursday morning 17/6/2004. My mum rang me and said, "Don't worry, if it doesn't work out we will find another way. If not☐"

I stopped her there and said, "Don't say that, and don't worry I'll be fine."

She said they'll be all praying for me

And I said, "Not to worry. See you after it's done."

I got off the phone and texted everyone who wanted to know, and told them the story, then turned off my phone. Then the doctor came in with the form for the operation for me to sign. I signed it there and then, and was wheeled into theatre again, and as the mask was being put on me to take a deep breath, to put me to sleep, I said, "This is it. Fix me up".

All I can remember after that is waking up back in the intensive care unit with my mum rubbing my arm while standing on my right.

As I woke up slowly, I had a completely different sense of life altogether that I had never felt while having the condition. I caught her hand and said to her, "It's gone"

I knew I'd never had a seizure again and, if I did, it was not going to come back like before. It was just like being re-born again even though I was in a total mess and looked like I wasn't worth a cent and drained from surgery and vomiting every time I moved.

But, at the same time, I just felt great and it felt so damn good that I even said to myself, I'd nearly go through all that again to feel as good as I do now. For once and for all, I finally knew I was done with that chapter in my life. I knew that I didn't even have to go back again. Just a few months earlier, it had also worked for Derry as well, who was a completely different person now too. It was more or less like my spirit opened potential inside me, and neurosurgeon Professor Ward was there as I could see him through a blurry vision. I put up my hand to shake his hand, and said, "Thanks."

That was the last time I ever saw Professor ward.

I couldn't stop smiling from then on and felt like I had a new lease of life. The anxiety, frustration, and negativity had all completely come to a halt, which was the best part of it.

I could finally look forward to normal things and see what kind of world we lived in.

As I was walking out of the hospital, a few weeks later, it felt like I was coming out of a dark prison. I saw and felt a completely new atmosphere that I had never felt before, that looked so simple. I almost fell to the ground from being overwhelmed by all of it. My aunt picked me up and I got into the car and shed tears of happiness, as I knew so well that it was all over. At the same time, I wondered what I would do with my life now after not having it for the last twenty-three years that is no longer possible. She replied, "Well you have the next twenty-three to look forward to." I laughed and said to myself, "Dam right, I do"

Just over a year later, when I was on the road, allowed to drive, I decided to go and visit the place again, not forgetting where I had come from. I went to visit the people who were in the EEG room at that time and brought Derry up too. The two of us visiting the two of them at that time had helped them a lot too. Just like Annmarie had come to visit me when I was there, who I still keep in touch with. So, I and Derry tried to give hope to the two, who were now admitted there, to show them that they were also on a road to recovery to their current situations and so on.

It is a massive weight off so much and very overwhelming to handle at times and the two people in there were so happy to see others it had worked for them. They thanked us for coming to see them.

Art and healing

I remember from when I was around five, which is quite a young age, that one afternoon I was up in Cork City with my mother. We had just left the hospital after going for a regular check-up, which was the beginning of a long series of events that had yet to occur. I was still full of spirit and didn't care about what I had anyway; it was harder for my parents than it was for me.

My mum and I were walking down Patrick's street. It was a hot summer day, and I saw this guy outside brown Thomas, painting a sort of Michelangelo painting and it caught my eye. I stopped and stalled my mum, as I was holding her hand and was fascinated by the amount of detail that was in it. I couldn't imagine someone's being talented enough to do something like this

I looked up at my mum and said, "Look at that! That's brilliant," and she nodded her head, laughing at how fascinated I was with it and didn't even think about getting home.

I couldn't take my eyes off its details, which included some kind of Celtic patterns, with people in the middle, and there were so many different colors and shapes in it. It puzzled me and nearly made me dizzy as I was looking at it. My mother had to drag me away from it, as I was trying to see how the artist was able to do this kind of stuff.

On the way home, I said to myself, I would love to be able to do that it looked so realistic and I never thought someone would ever be as talented

So, I made it my goal to be able to do something like that someday, and be an artist.

I didn't even try because I thought I would never have any of the skills. I was wrong, as usual, as I was doubting myself before I tried something, which wrecked my mind.

A few months later, my sixtieth birthday came up and my godfather, Paddy, got me a black Labrador pup. It was a big surprise. I was happy to go out, with him as my new mate. I decided to call him Penny since I remembered my mother used to have a pet dog with the same name.

Two days later, the next thing I knew, something tragic happened. The dog ran out the gate, all excited, got knocked down by a car, and was found dead just up the road.

I was just gobsmacked and more annoyed with myself for not looking after him, as I was responsible for him. Shortly afterward, we all heard the shocking news. Everyone went to his/her room to grieve the dog's death, where I was just sitting at the table in the kitchen, disgusted differently. I began to get my head around it all, thinking, Why do things like these happen all of a sudden, especially after losing Ciara recently? I gave myself twenty questions, thinking, Why did it happen so suddenly?

I just wanted to know why the hell did my dog have to die after a few days of living. So, while the rest of them were down in their rooms, all emotional, I became emotional in a different way. I wanted to bring the dog back in some way, so I picked up a biro, that was sitting on the table, got a piece of paper, drew a picture of the dog as best I could, and put his name on it after I was done.

I kept it for a while and didn't show it to anyone, as I just preferred to never be questioned and to be left alone at times like these. Eventually, when the dog was dead and buried, I threw it away, realizing this was another life lesson. These things probably happen to someone every day in some way or another so, after realizing that the sadness was slowly fading, I was more fed up realizing what reality brings to consciousness. The rest were really angry at me for not showing my emotions in the same way they did. I couldn't do so, because I was analyzing why it happened and was in shock before I got upset, and had also experienced something similar in a different way previously.

That was the very first time I began to create something on paper, and thinking about it now puzzles me. I do believe everything happens for a reason, and each lesson learned leads to another;

whatever road you take, good or bad, you always learn through it, as learning has hugely to do with your soul. It creates paths and journeys to help you aim towards your destiny or success.

From there on, I began to draw more and more using the biro, and I felt all negativity, I had picked up before, leave my body. I drew things such as animals at first, due to the death of Penny, then rock stars and bands playing live on stage. My imagination grew and grew the more I drew. I used to show my parents everything and they said, "That's great stuff. Keep it up."

I became more or less addicted to it, at one stage, and was drawing things every day such as faces, weapons, skulls, tattoos, etc. Every time I drew something, I'd show it to my parents. At this stage, they were sick of seeing my drawings, because I was at it so much that they nearly banned me from it.

All of a sudden, I got sick of it and didn't see it going any further. I got bored and completely stopped it for about twelve years until times became tough while I was going up and down to Dublin Medical Centre. Later in life, in Dublin, I had a lot of spare time at hand, and I was only beginning to get my mental health back after being depressed for years and losing weight and needed an escape from my current consciousness. I knew alcohol or drugs were not the way to go. So, I began to draw again after meeting Derry up there, who also draws, and to help me escape from reality, and to be able to look at something I've done without putting myself down.

I was always at this stage because I was negative, sour, and the consciousness in my mind from my depression had ruined me. I needed something to do as everyone does when they are leading up to a big dramatic change.

Anyway, I started by locking myself into my room, drawing tattoos at that time, because I loved the color tones and shapes. I read into their details, which were all illustrations and that inspired me to keep doing it.

I have an abstract mind anyway, and an eye for detail to see whatever the story seems to be behind it. At first, I drew things like birds, since I wanted to be free, and lorries, because I loved being on the road and I kept this up for about a year.

Flags and fonts followed this. That led me to more complicated things, such as Celtic knot works and designs. I worked on that for about six months, because I was fascinated by how all the knotwork was connected and how easy it was to create once you learn the tricks. It greatly helped get my mind back into shape. After filling books with pictures, I began to design my room in Celtic knotwork, and other designs like skulls, faces, and Chinese dragons, which I did in about three weeks with charcoal. It was all a way to express the feelings I felt back then.

When I was in Dublin Medical Centre later on that year, I met Derry at the E.E.G room, where there were only two beds in Ireland for this test. He was in the same situation as me, with the condition of uncontrolled epilepsy, and also was an artistic person from Cork. So, a connection was made, and a friendship began, that would later help us pull each other out of our respective mess using our experiences.

I had a small sketchbook with me to keep me occupied in there. I had a few drawings in it, and after hours of talking, I showed them to him. He was surprised and said that I do have the ability. He urged me to go further with it, as he was well ahead of me. He had been painting for about ten years, where all I'd done was sketching. He asked me if I ever tried painting and I said, "No, I don't think I'd be able to handle that."

He suggested that I give it a go and never leave it considering the ability he had seen in my drawings as he did a lot of it himself. He also explained that he had tried to recruit his consciousness to become normal after years of negativity, due to the structure of our current health system at the time. The effects of his medications kept him indoors for a very long time, where I was the opposite.

Art can be a great help in expressing your inner thoughts, building self-confidence, and the needs you want from whatever situation you're in. Maybe that's why a lot of people are studying it today: for its expressions, rather than as a living. They want to find a destiny for themselves, which includes happiness, rather than being rich.

Because no artist is in it for the money. The love of art is born through the nature of the artist, which includes the desire to be successful and not commercially inflated.

It took quite a while for me to start painting, as I still wasn't that interested, and was a little stubborn to start. Until one day, I met Derry when I was back in Cork City and he brought me to his house, which was not far from my place, and I walked in and saw paintings all over his walls.

It was like walking into a gallery, and right away, his paintings expressed how lost I felt in my skin, after being sick for so long, with no one to fully understand me. It was dramatic how I simply understood the paintings he had, and that made me see art in a completely different light.

I was impressed with the saturation, dampness, and lack of humor in the paintings. I asked him about them and each story he told me explained why each painting was in a particular category.

I was happy to find myself getting drawn into this conversation because I understood everything, and began to see how people talk about paintings, as before I used to think they were only made-up stories.

A few weeks later, I was up in my room and looked at one of the big Celtic designs I had done in charcoal. I decided to go over it with paint. It didn't interest me at first, and I found it so boring, due to the lack of color I had, but then I began to go to galleries, looked at different types of works, and also began to see that there were so many different types of paints for so many different materials. All of it created different types of emotions and structures and even stories.

So, I started to buy some paints. The first type I used was a critic, which dries fast and has numerous colors. So, I began to paint on wood at first, which I enjoyed and I did things like tunnels with blended colors matching from all sides, which expressed how I was coming to the end of a tunnel, knowing that soon an operation for my condition will take place. Also, I made a big Celtic cross out of plywood, with many colors in it, and cut it all out with a chisel in the end.

This was basically to express the end of one way of living. I got bored of that for a while because I had it done in a few hours. It was my first time working on wood, so I started to get canvas boards to paint on them and began to do abstract faces and shapes on them because I was surprised by how quickly the brush could glide with the paint on a canvas. My mind was abstract, and I believed anything could be created on this.

But, I was still drawn more to wood due to the shine it brought, but stayed more on canvases, as they were lighter, easier to carry, and quicker to paint on. Then, I began to get books with pictures of paintings. My style, more or less, grew towards Picasso, with shapes and abstract. I felt that I was at the right level for that type of painting, and began to look more into his works. I liked the way he had faces with so much expression on them that it made me wonder how his mind worked.

Shortly after all of this, I saw an option. I could do a course on it, which was signwriting. So, I went into the jobcentre in Cork, downloaded a copy of it, signed up for it right away, and my instincts said, This is something on your path.

So a few weeks down the road, I went in for an interview and showed him all the drawings I had done and told him I had never studied art but had a big interest in this particular topic. Then, he asked if I had the time to do it for six months as it is five days a week and full-time. I put my hand behind my neck, scratched it, and said, "Yes and no!"

He asked, "What do you mean?"

I said, "Well, I have a condition at the moment and am waiting on a call to get surgery, for it to, hopefully, be gone."

He replied, "Wl, that's not a problem. We have courses for disabled people."

I nearly crunched when I heard the word 'disabled', as I could never put myself into that particular category. But, at the same time, I expected to be shown the door, due to my memories in secondary school, which was nowhere near what I expected. So, I believed I was taking a big step here, but my instincts said, It's the right place.

He asked me, "What's wrong with you if you don't mind me asking?

I said, "It's epilepsy."

He replied, "Well, with the signwriting course, you might have to go up ladders and it might not be suitable for you right now. But, I'll put you on the list for next year, in case your operation has come by then."

I asked, "Are you serious?"

I expected to be just thrown off, as it was what I was used to.

But, he said, "Head off home, and once you have the surgery done, come back for another interview."

I said, "Ok," and thanked him for being somewhat helpful.

Then, I rang Derry and met up with him saying, "I think I got it but not till after I'm cured."

He said, "Congrats," and we went for a drink.

Then, about six months later, the call came, and I was finally cured.

Two months after that, I went back for another interview, looking like a completely new person. I met someone else in there that time and told her the situation.

I said, "I was here before, but I wasn't suitable for it then, but am now cured of the condition I once had."

She asked, "What was it?"

I told her.

She was delighted they could do such things then, and said, "Yes, your stuff looks great and you'll be good at this kind of thing."

The person I met the first time in there came over and shook my hand and told her, "He's fine," and shook my hand and said, "Congratulations!"

I nearly cried with all the years of being let down in secondary school. I finally had an option I want that's open right after another.

I was clueless about The fact that I had a massive burden off my shoulder, didn't have epilepsy anymore, and how fast things were turning around. I was an emotional wreck feeling overwhelmed, but in a good way for good reasons.

As soon as I have done this course, it began to open new options of creativity for me. On top of that, I loved it and didn't want it to end as I already knew how competitive it was in the real world of work. Learning this became a better type of environment for me to be in, as it had only been six months since the operation in Dublin. I was told to take a year off.

I created stained glass and did a little work on it as well as a few paintings, which looked very much like the stained glass. To be honest, I liked it. My favorite type of paint to use was American shot signwriting enamel oil-based paint. It just followed the brush and was smooth to use. I didn't like the a-critics so much anymore, because they dried too quickly, and were way too expensive to buy as a hobby. I had to be making a living to keep buying them off the shelves.

In acrylics blending, colors can become a problem as they are water-based. The saturation effects can be too light or dark, but not blended to the style I was into, so I decided to stick to oil, as that created a perfect structure and lasted a lot longer.

I and Derry used to meet up to talk about art, give each other tips and ideas, hit the galleries, and similar kinds of carrying on. He had been cured seven months before me and had the disease for thirteen years straight, so we were both on the same path looking for new lives to create and get over the burden and depression we both had experienced for many years.

I learned how to do different types of lettering, marble effects, vinyl, work on glass with gold leaf and gained computer skills, so it was well worth doing.

As that came to an end, I began to paint more and more on wood and canvas. I began to do things like eyes and handprints using bits of tissue, glitter, and other mixed media. At this time, I had numerous dreams, due to a new way of living. I had also begun a relationship as well, so I was on the right track at last.

The dreams I had were like me driving Lorries, high air balloons, and planes at full speed, where I was in full control. Some dreams I had came into paintings, so I was busy. I still have, more or less, that level of interest in art.

I joined a group down in East Cork later that year and urged Derry to join as well, and he did. I believe, our stuff was well-matched, but wasn't understood and stood out different, so I decided to ask Derry to join, as they were looking for more people. We had a few exhibitions and both our work fit together but was still so different from the rest, which more or less consisted of landscapes, where mine became like Derry's with meanings to them. So, I, and Derry, decided to take a break from them.

Now, I'm going to move on to another talent I had from a young age, which is writing. I remember at thirteen years I had a pen pal in west Cork called Shiv who I met in Cork Medical Centre when I was in for a change of medications.

She was getting her appendix out and we became friends very quickly. We used to regularly write to each other from each side of Cork because there was no such thing as the internet then.

I fell out of contact after I began to go to Dublin with her. But, I have relocated her nine years later and am also back in contact with her today. So, I used to write to her regularly and also send her the odd drawings. We used to look forward to getting each other's letters, as technology was scarce back then, and something coming in the letterbox was like a big surprise anyone is looking forward to.

When I lost contact with Shiv, at age twenty, I met another girl online called Maria, from England, who also had a condition called 'cerebral palsy', and we became good friends too. We were able to link each other's stories, no matter good or bad, and she helped me a long way during the depression and my time in Dublin Medical Centre.

I used to write to her regularly until mobiles appeared everywhere like crazy, then writing to her slowly stopped. But, then, one day, a local TD, who had just joined Fianna Gail and knew me from around, called me and asked if I'd write something in the paper each week since he had heard from people around the village that I was able to express well on paper about anything.

He asked if I'd write about what's happening in society today and how development should be expressed and other kinds of things down that line. I said ok so I did that for a while week after week. He would also write something on the same agenda.

One time, we exchanged letters, which was something to do with how the town and locals were behaving in terms of drink and drugs, and how they expect to live a happy life be-having like kids or people in general. I read him and he read mine and I remember they were so similar. He picked mine up and put it into the paper. After that, he said he got many calls about who wrote it, which I didn't want anyone to know, because I'm not the type that looks for points when all I'm doing is speaking my mind, so he stayed discreet about that, but mentioned that it was written by a young man who lives in the local area.

He said they were all complimenting how true it was, and that there should be things like this going on the paper more often for people to get a reality check and stop acting like they are looking for trouble because the community has nothing better to do.

I was happy about that. All of a sudden, I got bored of writing, just like the time I got bored of drawing, but continuing to write on the same particular agenda wrecked my mind. I wanted bigger things to do, but that was more or less how far that went so I packed it up for a while and it came to an end.

Until the time I met Shiv again, I had just begun to write again, as I was free and single, and had a variety of knowledge in my mind, from experiences of all areas, like traveling, being sick, the health system, and art and so on. This was when I chose to go further in life with it as my consciousness was always thinking of simple situations out of the certain faults the world had created.

After waking up to a new world full of experiences, I was not conditioned to the way we're made to live and began to view everything using my own experience, which felt like I was reborn in some way. And along with the writing for radio stations, like 96 FM in Cork City, emailing 2 FM in Dublin, and even going to the UK stations for a suggestion, I wanted my thoughts to be known, on how we're all manufactured to be monitored. We live stable lives using what we see on T.V. and how we acknowledge situations. So, after analyzing how the world had stabilized, I wanted to create more than writing to show people what we need to stop creating, like greed, and begin creating a world of knowledge and peace. My answer to that was community globalization, rather than forced financial globalization.

To do this, I went back to the art. I was probably studying maps for a year at this stage. I began putting countries on canvas and my first one was Ireland, in which I separated all the counties. I splashed them all on the canvas trying to show we're all one, let's just get on, and stop the wars, like the troubles in Northern Ireland for so long and so on.

Then, I began to look at bigger things such as the continents. So, I went to the drawing board, separated all the countries in Europe, and put them all on a single canvas, spreading all angles. I gave them their colors and joined the ones that were in the European Union, and half joined the rest that would have to join to create more stable connections rather than poverty.

When I had Europe finished, I did America, in the same situation as Europe, where Europe had a few countries on top and America had stated, because poverty still is in the background along with homelessness and emptiness.

Then I did one of the worlds, that compared all the poor countries to only a few rich ones. Due to our population, we are so out of track with what's going on in the world. We should begin to stop the wars and create a whole new development for each nation in terms of demands the countries have and refuel the world with the structure instead of empty promises. This needs to be done, day after day, by governments that are controlled by few elite psychopaths.

This art became common for me to do as it brought a massive awakening inside me later on and was the reason why I was so attracted to doing such art with maps. They all had a political meaning, where, while I was doing them, I was not sure what I meant, even though later on they made much more sense like I had been able to connect with my subconsciousness.

GLOBALISM

It was a miracle and blessing in the end that I learned throughout my childhood. I was absolutely over the moon and on another mission. I was no longer sick, no longer had to meet people worriedly facing similar conditions, and no longer had people concerned about me.

I no longer felt discriminated through the role I played in society and no longer felt idol or hurt or targeted as someone lower than them, as realistically I can only name a few who were there to help me, due to who they were. Many people were there to see me in a situation way worse than their own, some without realizing it and some realizing it. Because, when people facing small worries see others facing bigger problems, they stop worrying about their matters.

I had health. So, I could now control my destiny, for the first time in my life, and I felt invincible. I made the solid atmosphere more positive through my energy. It was sort of like when I was a child and had it anyway, I was still positive, but this time I was accepted for overcoming it, and it was earned.

Wherever I went, I linked to a new atmosphere. I didn't think once of the past I had lived through as I had woken up to a new life. I had started to forget where I had come from, sort of like someone winning the lotto. I never forgot the people who were always there in my life before and just got used to enjoying life, which was a new experience at the time, with no criticism or shame involved. Even though, some people would still come over and look for news about my past rather than how life was now. I would just simply smile and say, "It's gone. That's it, forget about it."

I lost a lot of people with who I wasn't able to interact anymore, due to how life was going now. Maybe, it was a good thing I lost them if they couldn't see me be better. Maybe some of them might have received some enjoyment out of having the problem in the first place if they couldn't accept the fact I was now better and cured.

This is the same sort of effect people have on some people who are successful in business and hope that they later fail, and can't handle hearing that they are becoming more successful because of whatever is going on in their own lives.

That's the same attitude on why some people's lives never change and continue to have negative characteristics rather than positive ones! And, they would sometimes try and continue the conversation to generate some bit of negativity rather than positivity. I was always ahead of them in my thoughts and described the most positive things I could think of. I said that "I just woke up after surgery like a new spirit had flown into my system and, ever since, I don't even analyze the past like I used to. Now, I know it's over forever and will just be a part of my life-path."

Anything I viewed, thought, felt, was now positive as I felt a new and wiser I was beginning while the old and shattered me was now being destroyed, like me, I was inside was now finished.

For the next year, I was just on a high, where I went back to college to re-educate myself and did a course in signwriting that I loved and flew through it. A few weeks before that, I had started a relationship with a girl from another part of the country. We moved in together a few months after going out together, so everything was just going great and life was blissful.

After finishing the course I had taken, I went to another college to study graphic design but was more an outdoor person, and computers at this stage bored me. So, this I knew was going to be a challenge. I stuck this out and did not like it as much as signwriting, but understood that there was a lot more competition in it for the long run, due to incredible demand for websites and so on.

After this course had finished, I had been off for a few months and was starting to get bored again. My dad rang me telling me he knew someone who was looking for a painter decorator and might have a lot of work on if I was interested.

Of course, I told him the fact that I had nothing on but a lot of experience. I jumped at that opportunity and said, "Yes, I will, thanks."

A few days later, I met up with Jim and spent the next few years working for him. A building boom was also starting in Ireland but I saw right away it was also a massive false boom.

These next few years, after I reached the limit of all the occupations I was in, and done all the things I was not allowed to do before, like driving and so on, and pretty much drove all over the country at this stage, I began to get bored and felt like it was not right to live like either.

There are still people in the conditions I used to be in, and that's where I came from at the end of the day. So my view of waking up, and seeing how the world works now, after a few years, was slow when I started to connect the dots with systems and countries and so on.

I'm going to start by explaining how I saw the illusion of success behind the falseness of corruption orchestrated from the very top of international systems down along with international corporations.

Does it ever really matter how we have to become successful, once we can be successful and regulate ourselves and not live this big concept of greed that will never be one hundred percent fulfilled?

Because, it is an unfulfilled characteristic anyway, orchestrated from someone feeling insecure within themselves, and having everyone acknowledge them when they've made it successful financially, or through illnesses as I have. This is not a path that lasts forever, as it needs to be maintained for someone to stay in that position.

If anything, the people who are successful financially are the financial slaves within creating systems, like I was emotionally when I was sick. So some of them, due to incredible responsibilities in societies, have a big thing in common with someone who is fighting for their lives, but knows what matters in life, and why is it both want to be left out of the picture?

Nobody does, because they don't see the point in trying to fit in with all the commercial false behavior, while their lives are very, very real. The language is fake, along with the commercial egotistical sensitivity, which doesn't meet the requirements of the competitive world. The rich have been in the game for too long at the top of every system, and understand the illusion and falseness of it. So, they are either trying to seek enlightenment or if they go by, their lower selves are in danger of being run over by incredible greed and destruction.

The fact is that greed has de-sensitized us towards our-selves; rather than existing in a society, all we want, in the very end, is final respect. Greed has developed us to believe we're being respected. In reality, we have just made the world more fragile and abusive. If we were to continue this system without looking back at the mistakes, we have made our children and our grandchildren live in much worse conditions, than the ones we are creating for the current middle and poor class.

We will all develop Third World countries leading to massive poverty and crime due to our knowledge of real problems that have been developing since Christ that can only be felt, such as starvation, corruption, torture, rape, religion, and war.

We should always orchestrate the knowledge that war does not illustrate peace, and if anything, it begins one war then another one and then another one, and will never industrialize or regulate a union, unless cultures utilize civilization, and world peace becomes our new world order, rather than greed, nuclear military, and quality of life.

The fact is that the Great Depression, followed by World War I, World War II, and another financial breakdown in the banking system, has ensured that the industrial world cannot be considered safe in few parts of the world. If anything, it must be made global and united to open more options and developments, due to our increasing population. Decade after decade of young versus elderly is happening, and the elderly are living a lot longer, even though corporations are doing some serious de-populating.

Each decade, since the antibiotic has been found, there have been one billion births. This is rising continuously, so realistically, for someone whose seventy years of age, the world's population has been created in only that length of time mainly in Asia with nearly sixty percent of the world's population.

This is astonishing as we're told that there is not enough food to feed four billion people. As we know it, to live the quality of life we want to live and to make peace, we have to consider unions working with each other, like the United Nations.

We should be forced to face certain facts that make systems work on levels of respect and not illusions of competition, economic destruction, and greed. Today, we have proven that we all think and want the same things, which do not include war and terror and do include knowledge of why we're here and respect and peace for our locations and families.

We have created sports, which show civilization has its place where we can all get along if we want to with some similar interests. We created a world media that has formed a global culture for us to believe and live by but was later obviously manipulated in many ways due to its power telling us complete lies for its power and greed.

We have created a transport system, where today you can travel many ways to anywhere in the world at any given time. We have created mobile contact worldwide, which has evolved the same as the transport systems. We connect mo-biles online. I believe it was when mobiles began, the world boom began, as there was an increase in demand globally and created, and manufactured people's ideas to reality and ideas became needs worldwide.

We have a final equal organized developing structure worldwide that every country benefits from, but the more we demanded, the more of our power we gave away and left corporations to get bigger and bigger. First, I think the way we have always treated one another especially in cities is rotten and wrong and simply a road to hell. We cheat on one another whatever way you look at it. I mean this in terms of finance. Some women will target men with money, looks, or materials to gain something out of them for themselves. Men will target attractive-looking women to gain confidence for themselves and to feel they have it all made, where really they only have it all bought, and live no differently than a lustful person could dream.

But, deep down, all we're doing is commercially acting like that and using one another for what we want in this un-organized world. Everything is not equal, and the more we see ourselves becoming demanding.

An important thing comes last, and childish behavior comes first until we gain something we have always needed rather than wanted. Then, we learn what it's like to not have what we need rather than what we want. We are all in this world to organize it and develop it into an easy-going environment-friendly place and not to eat out of each other's pockets and destroy each other's feelings and kill each other's families eternally.

Men can destroy women by cheating on them, smacking them when they are unhappy or driven by their lower selves and it still happens today behind closed doors anywhere you go.

Some woman gets into a bad situation thinking if she had a child, it will change everything for the better, where it will make everything more stressful at first, and dramatically change the person for the better, if she is a good person by hers nature and was on the wrong path due to feeling unfulfilled.

Women also deliberately get pregnant sometimes, even though it takes two people to create a pregnancy. But, while currently, the system in other countries is better than their own, they use better systems as an advantage, thinking that they are financially sorted, where it is only the start of another life that involves more responsibility. Some think if they do such a thing, the man will have to stay with them then. They will not feel insecure like they did before, where a man, who is surprised as he had been safe, feels like he has been cheated on and low. The woman ends up seeming less loyal to him than she did before, and he questions whether she deserves his presence.

Why doesn't government split these types of people up into different environments? Why not have them renting for a few years and keep an eye on them for the first year or two? If they're in a warning phase, where everything's going fine for them, then the government can offer them a rent-to-buy scheme for fitting back into society in the right way and living using the right standards. Even though government means mind control and the world's government would mean world mind control, which is always a possibility now with the way they have us do such things to each other compared to before. That would take the money they have spent on rent of the value of the house and, from here on, they are paying an affordable mortgage off, and have earned their way of living and can feel better in themselves. It's simple, and both will gain, and if that doesn't work for them, it means they are too stubborn or selfish to change their life direction. All you can do is simply put them into smaller places in smaller environments where they will have to earn their way with their system of choice. Since they don't want to fit into any current systems available, this will make them more motivated to get what they already had in the first place when they were in a perfect situation that they took for granted.

The biggest problem is that the governments who are in control for too long become desensitized, and some are greedy, and we all look up to them for structure. We need to also be the gainers to succeed as a society, just like they have to, as a government that works for society, and not the other way around.

I am just sick and tired of seeing so many people flush everything down the drain because they are not motivated by anything going on around them. They get depressed or lose interest in everything, not knowing where to go or what to do. Their lives just come to a halt. They become numb and live on the edge as if this is as far as I can go with their lives, and don't understand how to get to the next level or the bigger picture. When you reach that area, you, more or less, are in a motionless situation. But, you're not happy, because your needs may be, more or less, only short-term, but your instincts will remind you that everything comes to an end.

If you are not going to start activating your mind to create a successful way of thinking to be happy within, then you might as well think of throwing in the towel of pitying yourself right now. Because you are only living on borrowed time until you face the fact that it's time to change your ways of life and you're the only person who can create that path.

We need some serious amount of job creations and must work on demands that would suit our needs in a good, and environmental, situation, but, also, we must regulate people who have these abilities.

Here is how I see the world now.

I see America has been the structure of the world since the nineteenth century as it is the top economy. it loves to work for success and gives everything a shot whether it fails or not, so I think it can be focused, on being the local structure worldwide, but the corporation also has way too much power there and success.

There is like the superego, which means super false self that people rarely have time to conquer. And, as for Europe, I think it is more situated in an ideal location of the world where so much history, along with so many revolutions has come from. It has top destinations and so many separate cultures to offer. But, they are now being destroyed throughout the EU integration system, where people from other countries get treated better than in their nation.

This is not right, as people should be allowed a better life in their nation. They should not be forced to go to another nation that doesn't even speak their language. This, I believe, is destroying cultures and forcing us into a federal Europe which was always been the plan since WWII. But by who, is the question. As long as the bubble continues, the people act like sheep and never wake up to it all, just like I acted after I got better, but decided to change my way of life again, not forgetting what I was once put through.

Asia is the most populated continent with many idealistic ideas and amazing tourism and food industries, and if anything, due to its large population, it should be the continent in charge of any population problems and how to deal with it rather than countries that can only look after their dues to not being overpopulated.

I'm now going to describe how I see us humans, who are, individually, the most gifted animals ever, with so much to offer and so much to also take. We created a world because we are so intelligent and we only get bored when we don't activate our minds.

Money creates circulation in society's multi-circulation. In multi-cultural, society's work creates structure in life's purpose and makes a person feel better about himself/herself for doing good

But then, in the long run, we put money first and people last if we are unfulfilled in the current situation we are in, which leads to discriminating one another and comparing one another until someone, or some larger system, comes to offer better direction with fewer corruption and more global demand.

Corruption and so many people fell into the fact that they need so much in life and borrow, so much and the governments grabbed every bit of cash they could. They came up with so many strategies to take everything back off people's things, as though this will lead to another depression, if they keep going the way they are going, with quality in their lives and societies declining.

Structure creates power, but when greed gets in the middle of maintaining that structure, everything is credited and capable of collapsing the entire system. This is because only so much greed can be obtained due to going from inflated to multi-inflated. Everyone has the possibility of ending up with nothing, which is completely self-inflicted.

What we need, that will be the only option to get us out of a depressed world, is a one-world system, like money, but nothing to do with elite power or corporate gain and treat-ed, like cleaning the environment worldwide and regulated to that standard and not profit standards, the internet, weather. That regulates countries', and continents' behavior, to be able to learn from each other and teach each other for the right reasons and not for power. And, there should be males and females in power globally, to teach each other, just like we know males are providers, and females nurturers, but completely out of balance today in doing it like that.

Up to now, for the past forty-plus years, it was all communities we grew up in. This was the way of living for many of the last generations who changed the world from being modest to being competitive. Then, our way of thinking was very local but never forgotten due to that grounded culture. As time went on, the population grew worldwide, and more options became available to people, more developments became global, especially after the 9/11 attack in New York, in 2001, which the whole world heard about for another ten years even though corporations killed over a million in that time and not a word about it. Also, the European Union created its European systems, that involved so many countries together with separate beliefs and cultures.

It would have destroyed each other before this current project created world interest in all aspects and a world society developed from it too into a materialistic culture bar in the Third World countries. Of course, most of the developed world's societies simply forget about when life gets too busy in their own countries, and now television has it all; world cultures in it materialized into nations, along with the developments all in one machine and created global interest along with global demand for more programming.

The biggest problem with demand is the faster it grows. it develops greed and addiction. Greed is like a vulture, wanting more and more, starving itself to get itself its next fix of gluten. It never gets enough and is capable of destroying everything it creates.

People who never get a piece of the big apple are very ignorant to the fact they are not needed for anything with big responsibilities. They don't feel the ability to influence society's needs away from them on their behalf, so it creates moisture of illusion between the givers and the takers, and nearly always goes around in circles like an ongoing cycle.

If we're trying to create peace in certain countries then why in the developed countries do we create an illusion that to be something you must keep up with society or you're classed as a loser or good-for-nothing person who lacks be-hind?

Is that not the beginning of desensitizing people that lead to desensitizing societies, and if left, continues to be capable of creating privatized elites, who can do a lot worse than good for their interests without societies seeing if they are the ones maintaining the system.

However, the mind can be powerful, the internet has created a global multi-consciousness for everyone's beliefs and interests to be argued upon sharing their opinions on everything think of, I think that the whole world itself wants one particular thing: which is protection. America is the first to demonstrate that going to war most of the time turns people's beliefs into false hope, and false wars to build up coun-tries after shattering them and gain profit from them by running them their way.

To demonstrate this, America gave the G-TWENTY a taste of quality and success by teaching them the American dream and illusion. Everyone thought it would never end. The real leaders in this world are the Third World countries who for what I believe, are the only people who can survive and adapt to major lower living standards to fulfill their simple needs like feeding their family. They are true leaders of what the human body can adapt to, and create happiness by just breathing and being alive and keeping their beliefs.

Money is something that we all agreed to use, as a tool for needs, but got more powerful when wants came before needs from being unfulfilled. It may get you what you want, but it will not buy you true happiness, but only illusion lifestyles, that are no more than a fix like someone who is hooked on drugs, which is never enough.

Poorer nations don't live that false lifestyle they love to survive, and try to keep active lifestyles to stay alive, and are a lot braver like hunters and fishermen and more open-minded towards options for structure. Yet, also having to pay massive interest debts to developed nations who completely ignore them or have a war with them and were supposed to believe the developed world is the word of God. The rich nations can only adapt to something that society will negotiate for, because they're already ignorant towards the nations in more poverty, due to their division in their societies, and become just as out of touch as some wealthy people can to a poor person when they are enlightened with wealth and power rather than experiences. More suicides are committed in developed nations in today's world than nations in more poverty who die from starvation, famine, or disease that was not decided.

So, what is wrong when one country volunteers death, due to mental states of consciousness or corporate greed and destruction. That desensitizes people due to their character and makes them feel they don't fit in with the current society. These humans who have their way of living are recommended as being losers or nobodies when they just don't want to be part of the society that is current. Society is not fulfilled, either if they can spot these people before something happens, or more positive people start making us all be losers in different characteristics. Some financial, some emotional.

But here's another thing. If losers make others jealous because they don't have money, then why are the elderly treated as losers because they're no longer working or retired? But, are the people who have the most money the ones who have finished their chapter in the career path?

It doesn't matter what people say so many others will always find something to give out about, and for each person giving outcomes another negative thought into the atmosphere. Same as for each idea to someone open-minded may come another chance to succeed financially, while another person at the other side of the world could be thinking the same thing.

What we need is a world community, not a world religion or government conquered by international psychopaths, that would have a better chance of destroying us all, nation by nation, culture by culture, continent by continent, and, finally, the globe that has about 200 trillion worth of debt and 7.3 billion people on it at present.

If people learn what a derivative is in the financial system, and how it's monopolized, the very same thing can be done with humans, and completely monopolize them, and have control over them all without them even knowing it.

I think it's better to build a world community, rather than any evil system. Because communities talk to each other and wake up, societies work off each other, but there can only be one elite like there can only be one empire because they feed off each other!

Social engineering

We as humans are the most intelligent and creative animals that have ever thrived on this planet and know that there are over seven billion of us, which has never happened in history with the planet's population doubling in over 30 years.

If people are still alive today, who have been around over 50 or 60 years ago, and the planet has doubled its population in fewer times, how can reincarnation exist when these people are still alive today?

I think that we are highly intelligent. We must stay active for our consciousness to stay even a little stable, because we have lower and higher levels of consciousness, that are unhealthy, and so structured for perfection in anything we choose to do and can be our own worse critics if things are not exactly like we plan.

We must keep them motivated healthily by just doing what we're good at or more to the point what makes us feel who we are and fulfills us to live our lives in peace and harmony. No one knows what we're in this world for and how to stabilize world problems from growing to equalize all of us.

If anything, we can reunite as situations in the world get worse, because they always do before they get better. The fact we all saw structure in the world or sometime in our lives is how we're all willing to change for the better, rather than go back in time to an offshore less manufactured destabilized corrupt world of depression. Today over fifty percent of the world lives on fewer than 2 dollars a day, and the few who are rich are only getting richer, as the majority are in the systems the rich created, which is, at some point, going to have to collapse too.

We have created a world of organizations of businesses to cater to demands. We have now created worldwide communication such as the web, television, and radio where most of us spend our evenings and nights watching and listening to what's going on in the world to what is true and what's not so realistic. It has created a world culture for all our beliefs to be in whenever we choose to listen or watch rather than debating ourselves person to person playing comparison when the ego can get the better of us in those situations.

We are also the most selfish, unforgiving, optimistic creature, as we never forget about our countries' past events and wars that have happened to our countries or people. We brag about, it, like our former enemies, and create an unwelcome atmosphere for them that creates more ignorance and arrogance and so on.

We forget it was a previous generation at war with us and not the current generation who are paying for the previous ones' wrongdoings. But, we also do that to our people if we're not happy with ourselves, and it goes on and on. We just see others feeling more down than us because we are unfulfilled with ourselves.

The former cultures we lived through were filled up with so much resentment from the past that we disliked seeing others get on with their lives and doing well, when we're being struck into a corner, not knowing where to take the next step. Because, realistically, the people who move on are the people who don't want to fit in with the current society and that's what it seems to have come to unless in general as a species we change how we behave.

Creative thinking is the only way to manufacture our thoughts to success rather than being told how to learn to stay in society or be a part of a team and be good. If anything, we all think differently, and are all on different levels of success, with completely separate abilities, and live ups and downs at different times of our lives. Some may argue that success or failure leads to the success of new ideas, which is true in my eyes but we have created so much junk and material. Some people who have so much don't have the time to use it while there are others in other parts of the world, starving to death, due to the way their countries run and poverty provokes them from seeing the big picture towards any development. It's disgusting and wrong how much the difference between the rich and poor societies are around the world because how you think is how you succeed.

If people are going to be on the brink of collapse from starvation, where economies have no growth, then they should be given a chance to live in a different economy, with the demands they live by and skills they have. Rather than die, especially when some countries have population problems, and need more young people while other countries have exactly that, but can't afford to keep them alive? India alone has the population of Europe below the age of thirty today!

While fifty percent of the world is meant to be under the age of thirty-two, while the systems we live by are by people way beyond their age and need to be completely restructured. There is nothing wrong with being rich, but as soon as it creates your consciousness to be more selfish and more in tune with your animal side to keep up with the wealthy people, rather than creating a system for society to maintain and the community to benefit from and so on. Because frustration begins to build up in poorer societies and forgotten communities, where today the only places where people help one another and not in a fake way are in rich countries. What materialistic societies do is whether they know the person or whether they will gain as much as they are given back, like a bank gives out a loan with interest. People get so worked up over this, especially sensitive people, and some don't want to be part of the world when they see us act like this which is understandable to an extent.

But, look back at history, and what they have done while being together then, like the Vikings, for instance, created ships and transported them to different countries and ruled the world in their way. Then, along came the Romans who created the roads and the wheel and we lived in their structure then. Then, the British came along and were the first union to be industrial and one of the longest unions around today, over 300 years old later.

My point is, we're going to keep relapsing in cycles, in this world, with more people coming into it. We can't afford to live in a false corrupt world of lies and manipulation anymore. We need an agreement with global laws and communications and desire for people wanting to be a part of it, for the right reasons, of course.

The communication is already there and the motivation is also there. People do want to change but don't know what to change into, because they don't want to feel left out or peer pressured into anything to pacific, because so many people today don't want to be here or don't know what to do with themselves.

The only difference between America and Europe for now is Europe has several languages that can create a little communication problem. but other than that, both continents work together learn from each other, and understand each other's structure. Europe has an unbelievable history to it.

We created so much in history that still stands but is now being run like an empire through the Roman Empire System. America has invented the most basic and highly advanced technology worldwide, such as the Internet, electricity, and so on. They have been the structure of the world since, but doing a business is simple and basic common sense, which makes investment possible.

It's not the knowledge that we need to overlook our careers. It's the basic understanding of living needs, which brings you to the next level of understanding that creates inventions to manufacturing to business. But, now America has got so big too and also owes so much that it has become like a British Empire system orchestrated from the world's financial capital, London, which pretty much builds many of the world's financial systems in other parts of the world.

At the same time, money does not create happiness unless you use it wisely. It creates more greed and inflation than anything and people who have it couldn't possibly imagine living a basic life again until they relapse themselves. But, believe me, they fear it so much that they feel overruled by how much they have and how they know too much manipulation.

Trust begins to fade in some terms in relationships for that matter their consciousness takes control and they think people are trying to break them or clean them out. That's a reason a lot of them stay single, divorced, or don't marry because their consciousness is way too active. Just like a bipolar person's is unlevelled as they are way too busy. Some can lose so much and have no problem with it because their consciousness is so active anyway again like bipolar people are that they see other ways of scheduling and rebuilding their situations again. But, not all end up in that situation; some live a good happy life structure all the ins and outs of whatever they are investing in, or know people who would fit into their projects, round them up, and the process begins.

The problem today is that everyone who wants to get to the top of the ladder does not realize they must fail numerous times to get there. They go and take out big loans get themselves into an awful amount of debt live life as if their already rich where in the long run all they are doing is living it on credit and borrowed time but they don't realize it. There in full control of whoever loaned them whatever they owe without even fully realizing it. And they are going to get into a shock of reality when things get worse as they have and what they've taken will have to be replaced whatever the case by them or by society or by numerous lives of following generations.

Governments are doing the very same thing with countries and on too much to understand and feel they also need to change, as governments work for the people. Not the other way around. They enjoy a comfortable lifestyle and salary paid for by the society so, just like the relationship I once had with Gerard, societies are now beginning to have with their governments control them rather than work for them until they start to take more power back. They become more educated to also take more action to solve problems rather than create them for themselves and be engineered into a false boom or bust cycle.

We had, and are more or less, living a life of comfort playing with the rest of the country's population. More young people are needed in politics with more ideas and more creativity than those who have served much time and are getting tired and almost looking forward to a comfortable pension. People with that thought process can no longer serve people for their best interests and needs. Many of them are more out-of-touch with the new generations. They are desensitized and cannot interact properly with those who need their help more than those who don't. Countries and continents need to learn more from each other to inflate society's needs and beliefs for the future and gain more respect and friendship and respect for each other.

That was never possible before.

But, now that we are engineered and most developed economies, societies, routines, cities, educations systems, and so on are all engineered, we should be able to re-engineer ourselves to be ourselves and make peace with ourselves to make peace with others. And not fall into the social engineering project that was invented in Frankfurt where the massive private

European Bank also is so even though London still holds the world's financial capital Frankfurt in Germany seems to be holding many titles with all that's going on in the EU project that could only get much bigger and engineered into a federal superstate the fact they already have it done with the currency.

So, it's a decision for Europeans to reverse these systems and go back to their cultures or enter them and fit into a European federal system. If it wants to lead as a global superpower the first thing it should eliminate is poverty. The fact fifty percent of the world must live on 2 dollars a day while many in the developed world give out about the weather or something they take for granted.

KUNDALINI TO REPENTANCE

At the age of twenty-eight, organ failure from Pyelonephritis which I was not aware I had at this time until 35 had triggered inside me an experience I always wanted yet killed who I was until this time at the same time like it was a death. I was reaching a place where I wanted to know what I was to do with my life, now the fact I had just lived my childhood like adulthood and already had amazing knowledge about how the real world works like we all want to know where we stand when we reach adulthood.

One thing I did know was I was not one of those entering the real world now after being indoctrinated through childhood like most people are at that age. If anything, I was retiring my way out of it since I had done everything I had wanted to do and challenged all the systems. I felt completely failed up to now and being in numerous jobs that no longer fulfilled me and took numerous risks in life already that were not experienced for no reason, and I felt like very few challenges were left in my life as I knew so much that was not yet been exposed. And I didn't feel a nine-to-five job would fulfill me either as I saw that was more controlling than the life I had before and could not do it unless it involved little manipulation so that I would not be living a false life - ego life. Also, after having numerous occupations and reaching their limits, I knew I was certainly done with the construction industry.

I thought hard and could see I had the skills of an artist or a journalist and have already done journalism in the form of map art and many more projects on geopolitical research of the globalized world we are currently living in. So, I looked into doing a journalism course as I enjoy finding people who think they are more clever and exposing the truth, etc.

Then, I looked at the media and spent about a year looking at the news studying all the different forms, and searched who operates them and controls them since I realized there were so many more important things going on that were never exactly exposed with the full truth. Then, I looked at more things like films that were a lot more violent than before and so on, and computer games that were extremely violent with swearing words and pornography that were never around before. Even soaps, for that matter, that had couples breaking up all the time and cheating with others and having children with others and so on that happen so much in the developed countries now that it was just constant programming. So, after already growing up and being aware of the pharmaceutical empire and coming through it, I became a better person.

I started to wonder if there were sick people behind this big programming media industry and came across a guy (who I won't name) who had his media empire and said to myself, If that guy controls the media, then journalism is controlled too. Sometimes, by a corrupt wage, and other times, by death if you expose everything like a journalist is supposed to do but a whistle-blower now has to, and can have their life threatened. So I started to write more and put things together and also said to myself, If we all became journalists, then there would be no such occupation as a whistle-blower.

I was also well aware that something very big was on the way that would probably change me in some way forever and blow away all the other experiences I had up till now. When I began to realize all of these things, it was because my perception was dramatically changing along with all my experiences in life — so far starting — to completely make sense now on why I was put through all of them. And I knew the way I was living in general was not the way I wanted to live anymore, since it had no value, little satisfaction, and I would get too bored too fast to live a random life as most do. The kind of questions I started to ask myself was, Who am I? Why am I here after all I experienced?

What is my destiny, which was always enlightenment if it was ever possible? Those questions continuously became a new routine, not to drive me crazy but to change myself dramatically. They created the same kind of turnaround as re-educating yourself does in general but only once that state of mind is accepted by you. You allow more and deeper truths and experiences to follow, the same as meditation allows you to fully have a free state of mind and detox your system. This was becoming more self-realization etc.

The reason I knew something big was going to happen was that I already had something big happen in my life before. Before that operation, everything had fallen apart, and that same sense of intuition was coming back again but in a much more dramatic sense completely. Even though this was seven years after surgery, you never forget a feeling that you once had before; this was the same as love.

Also, I presumed it was another sort of detox program that I had built up since I had the surgery and that I was beginning to change my way again since that way of life no longer fulfilled me. This was the case after realizing that society was just as enslaved as I used to be and same as I wanted to gain health before I certainly was not interested in playing part in this way of living either when people in societies are controlled by elites as much as I was by medications.

So, I started to transform myself to a new level of understanding that involved world programs and world societies and realized I had finished a learning period in been programmed at this stage and was freeing myself from been controlled or manipulated to think I was free when I was not all along. Also, certain things in the past that I never fully fixed, kept coming back day after day. These were the sort of things that I didn't feel were any bit valid in my life anyway, so I just threw them to the side. I thought they were of no concern anymore, like the relationship I had with Gerard growing up, but they were things I was being forced to fix and get out of my system to be able to move forward again and learn from them. Things like the people I resented that I thought I forgot but never forgave, which were now becoming harder to carry than ever before.

Also, theories started to come to mind like the thought that maybe the heart works as the mind and that you become emotionally intelligent by the heart and financially intelligent by the mind, which is a lot more manipulating so no wonder the world's the way it is when the mind runs it — that's the devil's playground. And then that expanded to things like if that's true, then why are we not educated emotionally if the world wants peace? So many other types of global questions began to emerge.

All of this was after I made a bold move and slowly went completely off all my medications. The fact that I no longer had the illness and was seven years cured of it, helped a lot. I decided I was also not going to be dictated by medications and will see if going off them again will create anything new. So in a way, it was saying goodbye to life, as I was on them for pretty much my entire life.

And each year, I went off one type; and in the end, I skipped days without them, sometimes weeks, and nothing was happening like the times I went off them before. When coming off them, my mind became incredibly clear, and my way of thinking was a lot faster than it was before as if the medications had been suppressing me in some way all along. But, in general, the surgery got to the root of the problem so I no longer thought I should bother taking these either, especially from the history I had with medications anyway. I came off them slowly, year after year, which was difficult, but I didn't relapse from them as I knew it was just detoxing and my mind had become very clear and free after coming off them. I went from 12 pills a day to only 2 at the lowest dose and could not believe the difference. I felt much healthier than ever before.

Then, I began to wonder who funds this pharmaceutical industry? And who is in charge of the education system that educates doctors or anyone else in the health system? And where are all these new disorders coming from or are they, in any way, even scientifically proven? And the more I looked into this, the more I saw it was like a business that grew into a global corporation, driven by greed. It works exactly like international banks do, engineering cycles of booms and busts all over the world. And that if this is the case, then there has got to be some form of manipulation in it.

So, I started to look at its profits and I could not get over it. The pharmaceutical industry alone has a research margin of the GDP☐Gross Domestic Product☐that equals the same amount of 160 countries put together. There are only over 200 countries in the world today with a meager 62 people holding more wealth than half of the world's population, which gives them just over a country each with people being their cash flow. There are also 500 corporations running bigger and bigger mainstream systems in more countries, deteriorating traditions, small local businesses, and cultural roots, deteriorating the developed world from the top down. It is turning them into corporate welfare states.

This also establishes that an entrepreneur is more important than a politician now, as a politician answers to them rather than regulates and dictates their corruption. When they go too far in corporate crimes and should be forced to go bankrupt, they are given more contracts to do business until the people who created the corporate crime completely deflate on seeing and realizing the bad they created. Rather than jailing such people or giving them more contracts for more projects, these types of people should be sent to Third World nations where people live on nothing.

They should have to live in much harder conditions and they should be made to use their abilities on developing projects while they are forced to stay there and watch while they sober up from the corruption they have caused in the developed nations. This would be more fruitful than just giving a sum of money to foreign aid or some other charity. The latter would have had no meaning to them other than being just a number, this would be the only way to deflate such people back to their neutral condition.

Also, on another note, everyone's body is a corporation when you look at the bigger picture, and whether you use or abuse it is entirely dependent on how you decide to live your life or how it's regulated, depending on where you live in the world. But a corporation is also a system and can only last for so long till it's high time for a revolution outside and evolution inside.

After learning that, I started to connect more dots and wonder who exactly were the people in charge of this, which of course would be the big oil industry, being the number one industry in the world yet also capable of creating climate change in the long run. The next big industry I could think of was the banking industry. So I started to wonder about Europe and saw that the power of Europe is the power of the European Central Bank (E.C.B.) in Frankfurt, Germany. Which is also the same city where social engineering was studied so I began to wonder, who exactly are the people who are the shareholders of E.C.B. along with the fed and the Bank of England (being the oldest in the world, with London being the financial capital of the world and the British Empire). And where's the proof that they even have the money they loan out in the first place since it's a private bank?

For instance, Ireland gets a loan of 80 billion from (E.C.B.) and the regulators in Ireland's banking system just loan it out without any discipline. When society was completely inflated and the current generation at that time was almost finished paying their mortgages off, it was time to get the next generation into debt to start the next 30-year cycle again. And it was also known that Ireland had oil and gas around its coast worth over 750 billion at the time. So to me, that sounds like a plan to deliberately get a country into debt to control it rather than upgrading the infrastructure, etc. And if that was not the plan, there would be more money spent on longer investments that have permanent inflation to sustain them. Like transport systems that link more towns to cities, more cities to cities, and occupations that are more maintained rather than inflated and no longer needed when boom turns to bust.

After researching all these kinds of things, the fact that so many people were living the dream that was only created out of fresh air in the first place, and they thought they were doing good for society and that it would continue, which is not possible when there were fewer than half of London city's population in the whole country, I used to shake my head and think I was crazy to think this way. However, I knew for a fact wherever something good happens in an upside-down world, there's a deeper agenda behind it. And the fact that I was in an occupation that went well for about three years and now saw dramatic change as the world's financial systems collapsed, validated my theory. I knew the company I was now working for would soon be in trouble too and I had been here many times before. I said to myself, Maybe it's time to look at life from a different perspective anyway.

I felt that this false boom cycle was coming to an end, it might have also been completely engineered for my generation to be put into debt to control them for the next cycle. So I wondered, has Ireland been deliberately put into debt? And is this G8 or leading countries' way of trapping Ireland into a situation where it will be impossible to get out of to get a percentage of the oil and gas reserves or resources and so on? Or is it meant to at least stabilize the whole country into a Japanese system that has a public debt of over two hundred percent of its economy but can manufacture some of the best technology in the world and has a very low crime rate? In addition, over forty percent of its population will be over 65 by 2050, so many of its systems will be global at the rate globalization has come together?

So, like in some contracts, you have to pay your way out of them if you want out like getting out of the European Union that became another form of the Roman Empire.

It became clear, overwhelming and sickening, why it was not mentioned on the media either when I never understood that the mainstream media was more a profit machine than telling the truth. That alone showed me the media must be either controlled or desensitized, especially the fact that the people working in R.T.E. (Radio Teilifis Eireann) were getting paid way too much to understand the country's situations and that they were far too comfortable and inflated to care either. It was kind of like some rich people who are well off are desensitized. But they are still the people that finance how many live at the bottom, which makes no sense at all.

I don't think financial intelligence should ever be run within a state where emotional intelligence is much more valid and more powerful. Financial intelligence is a lot more ignorant as many in comfort are inflated by a lifestyle. They are allowed to live whatever way they can afford to, never thinking where they're going to go when they leave this planet or the damage their enslaved character is doing to society in general. Yet many live on the suffering of the people with emotional intelligence who are living day today, which is great if it's accepted, but it never is when finance funds it. It's sort of like commercial relationships overrule emotional relationships in today's world, which are a lot less real and more demanding.

So going back to the system in general, I believed the answer to the situation was to keep people ignorant and egotistical, and maybe there was some agenda

319

behind that. So, I went to the E.C.B in Frankfurt Germany, and when I got there, I said to myself, The last guy that tried to take over Europe in this country was Hitler.

I wondered, Have a few people at the top just changed their tactic to do the same thing financially to control the next generation and build a federal European system with them all in it?

Like Joseph Stalin once said, "Give me one generation."

We don't even know these elite people who have built the whole federal European system up throughout over 60 years?

As I said earlier, this was what I saw and thought when I saw the world after getting healthy. I do think there should be an equal European system, but, without it being dictated, and for every country to be able to trade equally with each other rather than working in one state spending fewer and making more, and sending everything back to their home country. I do believe in a European Federation but not a forced one where we don't even know the people that are behind it all.

So after going there and understanding the way the financial system works, I said that's like creating money out of fresh air or banking our minds, and loaning impossible loans and creating countries to run like multi corporations and engineer them to go boom and bust. This would be the work of the devil in my eyes, which stated that maybe they are trying to create one European Federal Super-State in the long run after most countries are in debt that they can no longer payback and that Germany will maybe be the capital of Europe and so on. But these were just thoughts and I could never prove to be facts even though they made solid sense to me the fact I had grown up.

I went through the massive manipulation of the pharmaceutical industry that does this to our health only makes us believe it's all a massive healthcare system to make us more healthy and better where the maintenance of the system is much more important to them than making us all healthy beans. Because, they would be put out of business if we all were exactly that, but the fact many states in Europe were living different lifestyles and we can adapt to any level shows that if there was a European state, many would live below the life they had. Because it would be below the culture they had to and adjusting to other cultures while others would live above the life they had and corporately gain more profit from those who are trying to adapt to another culture. And, the language barrier would be a difficult system to live with too. Especially if others who had powerful jobs in other nations were transferred to nations where they didn't speak that language.

It would be like strangers in charge of systems, where their wage is more valid than their job. Cultures can be merged but not intimidated to be forced together. Ireland and England, for instance, fight for hundreds of years yet join a union later the same year in 1973 and are still very alike. But that's a long-term agreement being the Good Friday agreement sort of like the love-hate relationship I and Gerard had but finally came to terms with each other. And a European Union cannot be forced to get on until all cultures are respected and are all on the same level of agreement rather than forced to interact with each other in complete separate beliefs and ways of life in separate parts of the world living through completely separate systems. Where finance is the quickest way to force people how to live London is a perfect example of being the financial capital of the world and now forty-five percent of London are from other countries most been outside of the EU. And the whole population of the UK is now the Muslim population in the whole of the EU with some radicals not being trained to live in a democracy at all and conditioned to force their faith upon Europeans. And now one in seven people jailed in the UK are Muslim but jailed for what?

I have Muslim friends too and the countries they are from do not accept radicalism at all and are friendly nations that you would not often hear of in the Western world like Kazakhstan. The UK is always the first place to look at a system because it is more than likely going to develop around the world, a country's capitalism works because it creates a culture but a continent's multi-culture of completely separate languages and beliefs is economic warfare and cultural savage. The very same is been created in multi-cultures to super states but by who? Trying to merge this same structure into countries is a way broader picture.

We look at the USA, and we see only some of them live a great quality of life run by the one percent, but at the same time they work a lot harder, they have to pay for everything they learn they are a part of the United States and speak the same language, so can merge into the same system, with each other the fact they communicate the same language. We are a united Europe that is more of a divided margin where history goes back centuries.

There would have to be a European language or communication structured a European wage, a European belief, a European army which is slowly kind of happening called N.A.T.O.(North Atlantic Treaty Organisation), where its capital is Brussels, where all the laws are made in the European Union. But my theory is power corrupts, and absolute power corrupts, which is very true and explains how everything should be regulated, so those who are the shareholders of the E.C.B.(European-Central-Bank) could be so far out of their minds that they never have enough and want this to happen and will control it in whatever psychotic way they can.

I started to look at other banks in other countries such as Australia, United States, and saw they had one thing in common, Federal, and wondered who owns them. I searched the areas where they were, and for each bank, I saw on Rothschild avenue, I wondered who is Rothschild and saw that they were an English family of bankers that go back centuries and even funded the Bank of England that began the American revolution? This made me wonder if the federal bank in America is still orchestrated from the bank of England system in London that created the British Empire.

If it is, then that means the English run America that became a British Empire superpower and now the fact the English are also in the same union as Ireland. They must have a very big say in Europe too and understand the system better than most when it is possible of it also becoming an empire. This is why it was a good idea for the British to stick to their currency, away from the European currency, and when I went to Frankfurt in Germany the very same street was there by the E.C.B called Rothschild Avenue.

So, after researching all this kind of stuff, I was incredibly overwhelmed and angry at the same time. I began to get serious headaches knowing that something very big was going to happen to me now that would change my life forever. I was only 28 at this time and lived through the massive manipulation of the pharmaceutical industry that kills more people than wars due to its enormous profit-driven psychotic engine. I realized that the central banking systems around the world were a very similar system doing the same thing to national economies using people like derivatives are used and manipulated in a currency.

One night when I was sitting down inside as normal, I felt an incredible rush of energy firing up to my head as if it were an explosion of consciousness from the base of my spine. The best way to describe it is to imagine a 110-volt plug that we use on big machines or frequency programmers. Imagine a 1000-volt plug being plugged into you and that you were being electrocuted. I thought my head was going to completely explode. It was so powerful and completely out of this world, and I was thrown to the floor. It was as if when you say something to yourself that then became more sound and real and exploded like higher vibrations becoming a much higher consciousness than I had ever even imagined could be possible. The fact I was not grounded, I was not aware of what this even was. Then when I came around, I felt incredible bliss, which was just indescribable. People who physically saw me were worried and mistook it as a seizure and thought epilepsy was going to haunt me again, but this experience had just completely blown away all the years I suffered and carried having epilepsy.

Shortly after this experience, I started to get other experiences like out-of-body experiences where your spirit gets pulled up out of your physical body and you float right below the ceiling and turn around and see yourself asleep below on the bed. The fact I could see myself was because they say your third eye is open, which I didn't know anything about at the time at all.

It brings you to other dimensions of reality to experience other realities where I presume artists brought the idea of heaven and hell and so on. Lower dimensions were to experience lower realities that are horrible. Higher is blissful and just out of this world to even try to describe, as time doesn't even exist in them. Positive thought creates quality but the bliss was out of this world.

Over the next few weeks, I experienced five different dimensions. The first question I asked and wanted to know was, will the people who do bad things and keep getting away with it be punished since they manipulate and control those who want to do good in this world? Shortly after that, when I went to sleep that night, I was brought to this big black hole after again been pulled out of my body, which was just like a lower vibration but it was full of these creatures that were like vultures which I presumed were satanic demons. And this was all within a few seconds, and I felt I was able to move around inside the dream like it was three-dimensional but that I was paralyzed outside same as you can talk to yourself inside but not express it.

As I felt this punishment, creatures were attacking me, and my heart was getting an incredible punishment as if it were a dartboard or imagine feeling heartbroken and multiply that feeling as if your heart was being destroyed for you to feel all the pain in your life so far in one experience which had an impact on me.

This was the first night, and when I woke up, I was in shock from the experience, since I had asked a question the night before and it had been explained in a way so I presumed I was completely losing my mind but if I presumed that then I must not have been. Then I had experienced another dimension while awake. This dimension was a few days long where I saw bodies that looked half-demonic and half-human, and they looked astral, and a thought came to my head that maybe these are people who committed suicide.

As the weather was also horrible and that it never was bright and was just dark and rotten most of the time. I thought to myself that the worst place on earth, at one stage, where people committed suicide, actually has this whether that was in northern Europe at one stage, which stays dark for around four months of the year and this easily links to that.

This experience was also horrible, but, Hitler, who was the evilest man in history, had also committed suicide so this would say he was here and not in the lower one that was much worse with demonic demons where evil people should go and burn. So if Hitler committed suicide the evilest man in history then how could he have gone to hell when they say those who commit suicide possibly stay here and never enter a better world or heaven? Then after that, I was back here on the third dimension and felt back to neutral, which felt normal since I was neutral again, and a few days later, I experienced another dimension that was also here but more blissful and incredibly more mature and alternative.

The difference here was a time no longer existed, and you could do remarkable things like fly anywhere in the world for free at the speed of a thought same as an astral dream. More you feel it rather than think it. Its effect is like what you see on Star Trek or The Matrix when they disappear to other holograms or dimensions of reality. Then I woke up and spat out the same as I did after an out-of-body experience as if I had just come back to my body again and had telepathic communication, etc. It was a dimension, which the saying time flies when you're having fun was constant except there was no illusion or manipulation there. It was all free and blissful. And anything in the third dimension was just a lesson learned to be able to come to the fourth and experience it.

The fourth is where people no longer were sick because the vibration of the atmosphere you are living in there is healthy and not in any way manipulating or destructive. Peace has evolved and environmental destruction was no longer valid either as nature and humans united and made the world a place where it runs and engineers itself. We just maintain it rather than destroy it for self-gain and there were even things possible like waving your arm through a building or seen everything three-dimensional that is real in the third dimension. It is possible to go right through in the fourth and walk through as your consciousness is in a completely separate place from the physical plane it exists in on the third.

Finally, the fifth dimension was not so different from the fourth where it was even more blissful and felt like more of an orgasm dimension than living area and it would be much too blissful to even try and stay there to try and describe here in the third. After experiencing all these dimensions, I was exhausted from it but still saw it as more of a trip than an experience for the life I had already lived through. So this was me after having a near-death experience from the anger that was in me after the life I had been put through and going through these dimensions felt like a life review that had a long-term impact after the experience and changed me into a much better person.

Later, I started to even experience more that I didn't think I would have been able for at all, were a few weeks later after coming back from the cinema, something else was beginning to happen at the base of my spine. Sort of like as if I had just been tortured by a chiropractor or been in a car crash, and this happened for about twenty seconds but was a very new experience. I just sat there and meditated while it was happening. Then a few weeks later, I had the same experience again, but this time it was more serious as if it was some rattlesnake in me trying to shoot up my spine.

I wondered from the near-death experience I had just how I could now express myself much more clearly and not care about what I'm here to do anymore or question who I am anymore and this experience was answering all the questions I've ever wanted without me bordering to try and find the answers anymore. So after experiencing this, I could no longer handle crowds and the noise of a crowd would generate incredible sensitivity to whatever I was going through like a form of severe anxiety that I thought could lead to psychosis. I could feel their energy, good and bad, which was playing with my emotions at the time. I was getting rapid mood shifts like I was becoming bipolar but I knew from what I felt this was something very big and clearing my whole system to the fact I was also off medications for the first time in my life.

One thing I remember asking myself at the very start of all this experience was whether I was reaching higher consciousness, higher awareness, spiritual awakening due to all the experiences I have had in my life already. During this, I could not get anything done as I was overwhelmed and exhausted. All the energy I once had was leaving my system and I felt new clear energy was coming, like a new consciousness much bigger and realistic than the one we are told to live in.

About two months later, one night I was weeping as if I was saying goodbye to the world I thought was real. This night I decided to go for a walk and get some air. I was walking along a cliff, and I threw my arms up into the air as if I was now free and liberated and felt completely at ease very like the person in the film Shaw shank Redemption escapes from prison and does the very same thing. After this experience, I felt I was on a new path and became happier and more fulfilled from being myself rather than impressing others in an unequal world, which was the game in the world I was once in. And, I felt I was being fuelled up with love and that I loved everything, everyone, and so on and that life was just incredible bliss. The next thing that happened a few weeks after this was I was reaching higher frequencies and my consciousness could connect to some sort of universal consciousness where everything felt real and nothing I thought anymore had to be questioned twice. I believe this experience would not have happened if I stayed on the medications. And the fact it did happen, I have finally found peace of mind and found a life that I want to live rather than choose to live for a place in society. And, it was as if all these experiences I had during this spiritual awakening were a detox program to all the tension and negative energy carried from previous experiences.

And I had found who I am and why I am here due to self-realization. And have also connected with numerous other people around my county and country and the world in all different countries and cultures who had the very same awakening experience in their unique way, which simply explained to me again that I could not be any different from anyone else. And, even though it felt like enlightenment at the same time, I know if it was that then an old friend James, who I kept crossing paths with growing up, that his goal was always to become enlightened. I said it this is what it is then he must have also had the same experience so about four months after having the near-death experience.

I met him out of nowhere and he was laughing as we didn't see each other for years and knew we were crossing paths again for some reason. I shook my head and so did he and I said, "Kundalini?"

Then his face dropped with shock and he explained his similar experiences and told me I was an artist and thought many similar things to me about the world and said he could not handle the experience at all at the time but had finally found peace in himself and felt like he was reborn.

Then this grew meeting to add others who had it but were much older than me and from completely separate parts of the world. And the whole experience of the kundalini awakening itself lasted six years with me and had completely deteriorated everything I had learned up till then and many who I met at the start of my experience told me theirs were about five years which is also very like the left and right brain hemispheres connecting. This is how the world should connect like the Western world and Eastern world connecting through consciousness rather than former empire systems again.

This experience was very challenging to deal with and a lot of people can go completely psychotic from it. If they think they are ready for such an experience but are not ready for it at all because you have to face your demons your problems from the roots. You have to forgive everyone and everything that you experienced you have to try and ground yourself for such a massive change and be mentally and physically able for complete death of who you currently are. You have to completely give up on everything you have experienced and worked for and partly retire from the material life you live in because this experience is like being hit by lightning and right away you know you are a changed person forever. You just accept who you are and manage to deal with whatever comes in life from here on and could even lose many friends you have known all your life because of the change it impacts on someone who has it.

The cycle of my experience was as follows where there's a very old saying that, The truth will set you free. This also adds up to the number 23 which I was when I was cured of epilepsy only this list of 23 effects rather than years were the effects of this major kundalini awakening cycle that was much more powerful than anything I could have ever imagined was possible to experience in this physical world in a physical body. without going insane from the power of it. Especially when I was also having kriyas that are waves of electric energy that pump information from the heart to the brain and later give complete feelings of bliss and amazement out of this world so it is also important to meditate ten minutes each night while going through this unbelievable transformation. Finally, the phases of it were as follows. I hope this story has had an impact on someone's life path and helped them deal with some issues they are experiencing or might later in life.

1.   Insecurity

2.   Self-Hate

3.   Self-Guilt

4.   Spiritual Awareness

5.   Kidney Failure

6.   Self-Realisation

7.   Self-Acceptance

8.   Dark Night of the Soul

9.   Out of Body Experience

10.   Multi-Dimensional Experience

11.   Pyelonephrisis

12.   Seizures

13.   Feeling All the Pain You Created

14.   5d

15.   Seen God or Spirits

16.   Feeling Incredibly Secure

17.   Knowing and Feeling Your Purpose

18.   Self-Love

19.   Self-Respect

20.   Ego Death

21.   Peace

22.   Liberated

23.   Enlightenment

A Born again Christian trying to be one because if God created the devil and all these deceiving experiences are created by the devil then god is real and always superior to whatever deceptions come in life. But it is also important to test them to expose them so that you cannot be fooled or deceived by them and warn others who are deceiving themselves and others what they are allowing by letting this be their counterfeit godly belief because nobody who has passed has any connection here after death until God resurrects them from their graves. And this is from myself whose been far close to my own grave far too many times as it is.

THE EVIDENCE

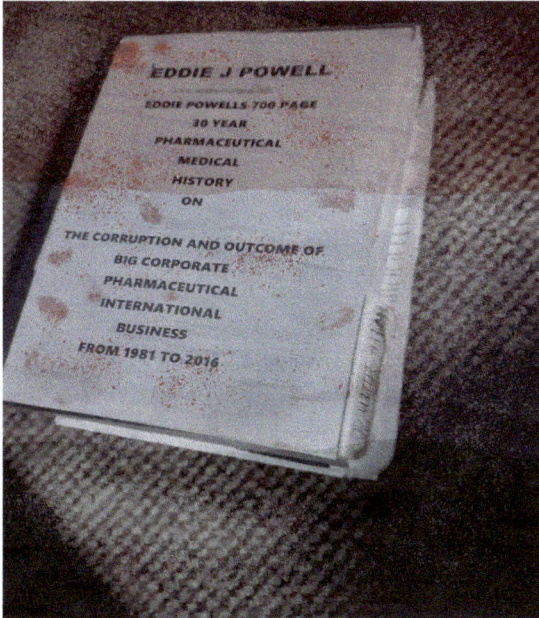

This is the document that proves every findings I have written in this work. It outlines the financial sinister plot that pharmaceutical and medical companies have been doing. These practices have proliferated for long years that a mafia can seemingly be conceived out of their practices.

Rather than cure, these mafia tactics resulted in some sickening outcomes. The sick is medicated with imbalanced medical treatments like a car that starts to break down when improperly driven. Living off the sick and unhealthy has become these companies' revenue system and those in it took all the credit which what makes the healthcare become an industry rather than race for cures model.